BUILDING A NON-ANXIOUS LIFE

"Do not be anxious about your life, what you will eat or what you will drink, nor about your body, what you will put on. . . . Which of you by being anxious can add a single hour to his span of life?"
—Matthew 6:25, 27 ESV

BUILDING A
NON-ANXIOUS LIFE

DR. JOHN DELONY

FOREWORD BY DAVE RAMSEY

Published by Ramsey Press, The Lampo Group, LLC
Franklin, Tennessee 37064

This publication is designed to provide accurate and authoritative information with regard to the subject matter covered. It is sold with the understanding that the publisher is not engaged in rendering financial, accounting, or other professional advice. If financial advice or other expert assistance is required, the services of a competent professional should be sought.

The names and other identifying facts of some individuals whose stories appear in this book have been changed to protect their privacy.

Editor: Kris Bearss
Cover Design: Chris Carrico and Weylon Smith
Photography: Seth Farmer
Interior Design: PerfecType, Nashville, TN

ISBN: 979-8-887820-01-9

Printed in the United States of America
23 24 25 26 27 WRZ 5 4 3 2 1

Praise for *Building a Non-Anxious Life*

"Everyone has anxiety in some form or another. It seems to be the defining condition of modern human brains. But until now, there's been no go-to manual that can help anyone, no matter their background, understand the science and soul of the problem—and also find solutions. *Building a Non-Anxious Life is* that manual. Its wisdom is wide and deep and delivered in a way that's empathetic, straightforward, and true. This book will help you unpack the deeper reasons why you're anxious and provide you with actionable tools that lead to lasting freedom."

Michael Easter, author of *The Comfort Crisis* and *Scarcity Brain*

"In this era where we have taken full ownership of anxiety being an inevitable default mode in an increasingly fast-paced society, I cannot think of a better book or better ambassador that might help us not just cope but conquer (and re-conquer) it on a daily basis than John Delony. I believe strongly that our purpose will almost always be attached to some level of freedom that others desperately need. John is walking hard in his purpose, gifted in being able to provide choices for us to make rather than negativity for which we have to settle.

"Being able to choose things like connection over isolation, belief over paralyzing fear, and even choosing the hard thing over the most convenient is giving us freedom from being resigned to a life that doesn't feel worth living. As a former advocate and spokesperson for youth suicide prevention and mental-health awareness, it brings me so much hope to know that information like this is being released into the world. This is content that will go far in giving us access to a better, more joyous, more stable quality of life. As John says himself, 'I would not have written this book if I didn't believe there is hope. For you, for me, for our kids, for the people we love, and for our world.' Amen to hope. May you find it as you read."

Jade Simmons, author of the #1 bestseller *Audacious Prayers for World Changers*, concert artist, and speaker

"Every time I've asked a mental-health professional to talk to me about anxiety, I've somehow left the conversation feeling *more* anxious. Then I met Dr. John, who has this superhero-like ability to be comfortably relatable when talking about things that have been overly intellectualized for far too long. This book is a celebration of everything that makes us human, a reminder of how beautiful it is to be perfectly imperfect, a master class on the healing power of community, and a road map on how to become our most fully realized selves."

Will Guidara, James Beard Award-winning restaurateur

"Not only has listening to Dr. John Delony's podcasts and reading his books changed my life for the better, but I am grateful to call John my personal friend. Not only does he have an unbelievably deep knowledge of mental health, but he has been transparent about his own struggles and cares DEEPLY to improve people's lives. Unlike many experts who talk in circles and do not provide clarity, John always provides clear, actionable instructions to improve your life. If you are willing to do the work, John's material will improve your life."

Dr. Layne Norton, founder of BioLayne and best-selling author

"John Delony's great new book, *Building a Non-Anxious Life*, is filled with crucial insight into the challenges we all face as we try to navigate today's hectic and anxiety-inducing world, and how to overcome them to build a better life. Through a combination of personal stories and insightful observations, John gives us easy, practical ways to create a peaceful life."

Dr. Caroline Leaf, cognitive neuroscientist and best-selling author

"In a post-Covid world, I am battle weary from the last few years. If that also describes you, then you too need to read this book.

"You will see a word that recurs often in this work: *choice*. Dr. Delony, to vastly oversimplify the beautiful messages in his book, has one overriding goal with this work: to give you back the choice that was so wrongly taken from you these past years. He reiterates a message I tell all my patients: All control is self-control. That's where it starts and where it stops.

"While Dr. Delony gives these messages with his usual humor, wisdom, and vulnerability, he is always clear that this book is not about his accomplishments but about yours. This book is about unlocking the person you still are, even in—and especially in—this brave new world we find ourselves in."

Michael Gomez, PhD, Director of Child and Adolescent Mental Health and Assistant Professor at the Pediatrics Department of Texas Tech University Health Sciences Center

"This book is an ice bath for the soul: a jarring yet essential plunge for anyone who suffers from anxiety."

Joshua Fields Millburn, The Minimalists

"John Delony is one of the few honest voices in mental health. His advice is authentic, applicable in the real world, and effective. If John says something, we always listen."

Sal DiStefano, personal trainer, co-founder of Mind Pump Media, and co-host of *Mind Pump* radio show and podcast

"Dr. Delony addresses head-on the sources and causes of anxiety and offers his readers remedies and paths to peace. Fear is often not our friend, and to have our feelings be our employee, not our employer, sets us free. Dr. Delony's work is a path to freedom and a life lived to the fullest."

Dr. Andrew Young, hostage negotiator, crisis counselor, and professor at Lubbock Christian University

"This book is so honest and relatable! In this book, John helps us understand the need to start the challenging but necessary move to build a non-anxious life. Our lives depend on it! His guidebook will have you taking notes in the margins and wanting to remember every piece of information he shares. So break out your highlighter and pen as you walk through this journey of regaining your life."

Dr. Lynn Jennings, Jennings & Associates Counseling Services and Texas Tech University Health Sciences Center

"Dr. John Delony has spent his career seeking ways to bring joy, peace, connection, and health to members of his community. He has relentlessly pursued new tools to sharpen his craft along each phase of his journey, and his book *Building a Non-Anxious Life* is the culmination of such effort. It is a masterful assimilation of the concepts from his first two books, brought together in a practical way to give his readers (and listeners) the tangible tools and steps needed to help them along the path of deliverance from the chains of anxiety."

Jeffrey D. Smith, MD, Assistant Professor of Family Medicine at Frist College of Medicine, Belmont University

For Sheila—

My light in the darkness.
My lifelong adventure.
My love.
My home.

For Hank and Josephine—

My heartbeats.
My deepest laughter, joy, love, and silliness.
My greatest gifts and my greatest mission.
My hope for the future.

For David and Addell Delony—

You built legacy out of the ashes of a great war.
You stayed married over 70 years.
You taught, held firm, laughed, and loved.
You gave me a road map for a non-anxious life.

CONTENTS

FOREWORD BY DAVE RAMSEY

I have anxiety. You have anxiety. Everyone has anxiety. The question's not whether we have anxicty; it's how much of it we have and what we should do with it. All you have to do is look past the end of your nose and you'll see someone struggling at some level with some amount of anxiety. Are they handling it well? Is it ruining their life? Are they out of control? Or are they functional? When I look in the mirror, I can ask the same questions.

The fact is, we are the most stressed-out, anxiety-ridden, out-of-control culture in history. And the paradox is, we have the most prosperity we've ever had and shouldn't be worried. Most people don't have to worry about food, shelter, or clothing, and yet all the despair statistics are up—suicide, depression, anxiety. Everywhere we look, there are signs of anxiousness, and it's ruining way too many people's lives.

Noticing this rise in anxiety in the past few years, we launched a quick read at Ramsey with Dr. John Delony titled *Redefining Anxiety*. After it sold hundreds of thousands of copies, we realized John had a lot to say to all of us about anxiety—how to define it and how to deal with it.

In this follow-up book, *Building a Non-Anxious Life*, John dives deeper. He brilliantly puts in front of us not just a compelling definition of anxiety but also the seven choices we can make to virtually eliminate it in our lives. I believe it's the best material I've read to deal with one of the greatest problems facing our culture.

As you'll see, John is not afraid to share his personal journey of dealing with anxiety. He's also not afraid to take a traditional, psychological-textbook approach to the subject of anxiety while simultaneously challenging a lot of the traditional, psychological-textbook approaches to this subject. The mix is refreshing and empowering . . . *and* will cause some people in the psychology world to struggle with his conclusions. Those of us in the *real* world, however, love his conclusions—because they're applicable, they're crammed with common sense, and they follow a strong intellectual construct.

The insight we get from *Building a Non-Anxious Life* isn't under the pretense that a *non-anxious* life exists. Life is not devoid of anxiety. Rather, it's understanding that it's possible to live a *less anxious* life by making intentional choices. It's acknowledging there will always be struggle in some area of our lives. Stuff is always going to come at us, and we have to deal with it. But the seven choices John outlines give us the ability to effectively deal with the inevitable onslaught of life's struggles and the anxiety that comes with them.

To the extent we understand these choices and observe them on a daily basis, our lives will become more joyful and more functional, and our relationships will improve. To the extent we follow these choices, we will experience peace like never before.

I'm excited at the journey you're about to start. You're on the brink of building and living a life you might not have thought possible. But building a non-anxious life *is* possible. And in the following pages, John will show you how.

INTRODUCTION

CANNONBALL

It's not hard to fall
When you float like a cannonball.
Damien Rice, "Cannonball" (2000)

The first time I ever took a call on live radio was in front of millions and millions of people, on the second-largest radio program in the country. And I had no experience in radio. Zero. I didn't know how to speak concisely, how to come in and out of commercial breaks . . . any of it. I was totally exposed, like the bad dream where you're giving a presentation in high school and you look down and suddenly realize you're not wearing any clothes. It was a call-in advice show, and I completely tanked my first call. I still remember freezing when the person asked me a comically simple question.

For the rest of the broadcast I was a spastic mess— sometimes my answers didn't make a lot of sense, and I developed weird vocal tics. One person called in to the show to complain about me, saying I was like a worm on hot coals.[1] But the train kept moving. And with some great coaching from Dave, James and the production team, and some of my other colleagues, I started to get the hang of it. It was a lot like changing the oil in the car while the car is flying down the highway.

This was in the summer of 2020, and people were calling in to the show about how anxious, worried, and burdened they were. It seemed everyone was anxious.

About Covid.

About the lockdowns.

About masks or no masks, shots or no shots, social passports and rising death tolls.

About the countless jobs evaporated overnight and losing their livelihood, their income, their sense of community, and in many cases, their basic dignity. And since millions and millions of Americans live paycheck to paycheck and have few, if any, relationships outside of work, people were anxious about their very existence.

They were scared about their struggling kids, crumbling marriages, how to juggle a second job as a homeschool

---

[1] I played the recorded complaint for my kids, and they thought it was the funniest thing they'd ever heard.

teacher, giving birth in the hospital all alone, or being unable to visit aging family members who were passing away. Millions and millions of people were told they *weren't essential*. Life was chaotic.

The world was electric and crackling.

And this wasn't a projection or an exaggeration. I felt it too. In my own home.

With no time for romance or connection, my wife and I quickly became co-managers of our house. I watched my kids get buried by Zoom school, and as someone who spent my entire pre-radio career studying and working with young people and their families, I was troubled by the disastrous effects this would have on their educational and social development.

I was also dreadfully lonely myself.

I could text and share memes, but I desperately missed my friends. And hugs. And punches on the arm. And laughing so hard I couldn't breathe. And in-person disagreements over hard life issues and who was going to pay for the chips and salsa. I was withering.

I did get to know my neighbors. We had socially distanced cookouts, driveway hangouts, and we picked up groceries for each other. But underneath the pleasantries, and after all the pivoting that life required just to get through another week, my anxiety and depression alarms were ringing off the wall.

Yours were ringing too.

EVERYTHING CAME UNDONE

Covid didn't give us all anxiety. It poured gasoline on a growing fire that's been burning for years. Depending on what data you examine, anywhere from a quarter to half of the US population reports their lives are affected by anxiety, stress, or burnout. Anxiety is everywhere.

Before we go any further, I want to make sure we're using the same language. When I say *anxiety*, I'm talking about all of it. Yes, I'm referring to clinical anxiety, phobias, and social anxiety. But I'm also talking about debilitating worry and fear and chronic stress and burnout, and how our lives have been flooded with constant, heightened levels of threats and chaos. Anxiety is no longer just a clinical term—it's now part of the cultural vernacular. It encompasses everything from panic attacks to feeling lonely, angry, scared, or buzzing from the low-level hum that something big and scary and unseen is coming our way. So for the sake of this book, instead of playing diagnostic word games, I'm going to call it all anxiety.

Make no mistake: Things *are* happening. Big changes *are* coming. Most of us *are* right to be scared sometimes. The world will always be changing, both in massive leaps and in bumbling, crooked ways.

But this is not why everyone is buzzing, anxious, and stressed.

We're buzzing, anxious, and stressed because we've created a world our bodies can't exist in. We weren't designed for digital yet physically distant relationships. Our bodies can't handle the countless pressing emergencies and life tragedies, the onslaught of never-ending global trauma, and the incessant bells, clicks, and dings of notifications, murder podcasts, online learning, and an Artificial Intelligence arms race all at the same time. We humans have never had to live in an endless sea of information, opportunity, mating choices, food, and mobility. It's a tsunami of both great and terrifying things. We just have so much . . . everything.

We're trying to stay alive on a concoction of cortisol and adrenaline and unearned dopamine, and as the great Dr. Bessel van der Kolk says, the body is keeping the score of all of it.

In this new world of *everything all at once,* we've missed the mark about how to respond. We don't know what the elusive "good life" even looks like anymore. Consequently, the things we've been doing to reduce or resolve our anxiety aren't working. Instead of freeing us to thrive like we'd hoped, our efforts often aren't even keeping our heads above water. We're putting band-aids over bullet holes. No wonder things feel like they're coming apart.

NOT THE ISSUE

One day while I was co-hosting *The Ramsey Show*, a caller wanted to know how to get rid of his anxiety. He was scared and had a lot of things going on in his life, and he kept talking about himself like a broken machine that needed to be fixed. After listening to him for a while, I finally told him, "Sir, with all due respect, anxiety is not the issue here."

During the commercial break, I took off my headphones and turned to Dave Ramsey, the co-host, and said, "Everybody keeps asking about anxiety. Anxiety isn't the problem. Anxiety is just the alarm system letting people know things are off the rails. People have created very anxious lives, and their bodies are trying to get their attention."

For years I'd been telling this to anyone who would listen—students, counseling clients, colleagues . . . even myself. Anxiety is just a smoke alarm, letting you know that something in your house is on fire. The alarm is not the problem. The fire is.

Dave replied, "You need to write that down. That's your first book right there."

And so it was.

In the summer of 2020, I wrote a 65-page quick read titled *Redefining Anxiety*. My friends called it a pamphlet. My mom called it a masterpiece. My young daughter simply laughed and said, "Dad . . . that's not a book."[2]

It was a to-the-point look at what anxiety is and isn't, and how to deal with it in both the short- and long-term. I wrote the book because people were hurting, and I knew that yet another scientific treatise on this topic was not going to help anyone. We all needed (especially me) a quick and simple understanding of the myths surrounding anxiety, the truths about anxiety, and ultimately, how to get our lives back.

---

[2] I'm learning in very real time that few people can humble you faster than a seven-year-old daughter with an opinion.

Redefining Anxiety took off.[3] The book touched a nerve and found its way into homes, purses, glove compartments, and classrooms across the country. I heard from counselors, psychologists, medical doctors, and business leaders who bought cases to hand out to their patients, clients, and employees. I heard from parents of teenagers, active-duty military personnel, and senior citizens. Everyone seemed worried about what was happening to their minds, bodies, and families. And most people were grateful for a new paradigm—a new way of looking at anxiety and what they could do next.

Here's the deal. I knew people were anxious. I knew because I'm always nose-down in the latest mental-health research, and because I have two decades of experience working with people in the messiest, most chaotic experiences of their lives. I'd also recently been traveling the country, sitting behind closed doors with construction workers, moms and dads, university executives, business leaders, teachers, students, and multimillionaires. I was hearing it everywhere. The world felt like it was burning down around us.

And for the first time in years, I was feeling that way again too.

I clearly remember being buried by my own anxiety: Unable to sleep despite increasing levels of exhaustion. Sharing a bed with the woman who loved me, yet still feeling completely alone. Paranoid that *Everyone is coming after me!*

---

[3] Or, like Gwen Stefani would say, "It was B-A-N-A-N-A-S."

or *It's all coming down!* while feeling the shame and despair of *This is my fault and I can't do anything about it.*

I talk so often about anxiety because I see it everywhere. I see it in my friends, my family, and in the mirror. I hear from you and how much you're hurting, and I remember how anxiety burned scars through my marriage, my relationships with my kids, my work, and my belief in myself.

And here it was, coming back from the dead, like a horror-movie villain.

A DIFFERENT KIND OF BOOK

So you and me . . . we're in this one together.

I'm not talking at you; I'm walking with you. I left out all[4] the counseling and psychology jargon and the endless theoretical propositions. Personally, as a former academic nerd, I find great value in theories and ideas. I believe they have their place in the world. But not here. They are great for contemplation and inquiry. I don't find them helpful when my friend is weeping or I'm sick to my stomach with fear and stress.

What you're about to read is not yet another pop-psychology piece or a work on how to be less anxious in the moment.[5] This book is exploring the foundation beneath

---

[4] Okay, okay . . . *most* of the jargon, not all of it.
[5] My book *Redefining Anxiety*, however, IS geared toward helping someone who is experiencing anxiety or acute stress right now.

the house. We're going to get to the root of the issue in a straightforward way.

As the world has become increasingly complex and chaotic, our biggest worries are morphing. I used to frequently get questions like "How do I help my son with his ADHD?" or "Can you help me and my husband get back 'that lovin' feeling'?"

Now people are asking, in quiet, wide-eyed existential fear, *"Will I ever be able to sleep through the night again?"*
"Has democracy run aground?"
"How do I stay sane in a world gone mad?"
"What hope can I offer my kids for their future?"
Everyone is anxious.

In the pages to come, I want us to address the root of concerns like these that have become such a part of everyday life.

And I'll also address hope.

As you read this book, do not forget . . .

This is a book about hope.

Hear me say loud and clear: I am profoundly hopeful about what comes next in your life, in your relationships, and in our world.

So if you're wanting information about diagnostics, brain function and chemistry, or the bio-social-physiological mechanics of anxiety from brilliant researchers, scientists, and clinicians from all over the world, I invite you to take your pick of the few million books, articles, and podcasts out there covering everything from anxiety and diet to anxiety and grief, anxiety and health, anxiety and medicine, and practically anything else you can imagine. But I've found that explaining the interplay between cortisol and epinephrine is not helpful to the exhausted single mom of three who can't get her heart to stop beating out of her chest. An elegant discussion about the HPA axis, serotonin reuptake and dopamine modulation, and an overactive amygdala is the least of worries for the over-the-road truck driver who misses his kids so much he can't breathe. Or for the nursing student who can't stop the hurricane of ruminating thoughts. Or for the man who finds himself yelling at the driver ahead of him for going too slow, too fast, or too whatever—he's just mad.

At the end of the day, though we're told the anxiety numbers are going up and up for everyone, everywhere, *anxiety is not the problem* for the vast majority of us. The fire that's setting off all the smoke alarms is the problem. And all our attempts to cobble together the right combination of podcasts, self-help books, prescription drugs, and bi-monthly counseling sessions in order to stay sane—or to even simply stay alive—are not putting out the fires. We're trying to float like a cannonball.

I'll say this directly because there's too much at stake: **What we're doing is not working.**

What *will* work is the real-world scratching and clawing for truth. And rediscovering the old roads taken by millions of weary travelers over centuries who, while moving from place to place, took their circumstances and created something a little better than what they inherited.

What will work is exploring the choices each of us can make, day by day, to create a more peaceful, joyful, and non-anxious life.

CHIPS AND QUESO

In all of this, I'm walking with you, not talking at you. I won't be lecturing you—I'm still figuring out some of these things myself. Think of this book as a conversation between you and me, over chips and good queso.[6] You and me, figuring out the next right step. Reimagining where we go from here. And what our lives can look like if we stop ignoring the smoke alarms and start fighting the fire with honest questions like:

"Why are my anxiety alarms going off all the time?"

"Why do I feel like I'm in an endless cycle of blame and anger and impatience?"

"Where did my addiction to comfort and avoidance come from?"

"Why are the people I love most melting down around me?"

I don't care who you are, what has happened to you, what you've done, or where you think your life is headed—it is never too late to change your relationships, your environment, your choices, or your life. And the change can begin right now.

You are worth making changes.

------

[6] Simmering with chunks of meat and good cheese and not just, as one of my favorite thinkers, Andrew Peterson, says: *orange cheese-juice*. Gross. Be better, orange cheese-juice eaters.

It's time to start solving for freedom. You will have to make choices, both simple and deeply challenging. But those choices will allow you to build something enduring and new: a non-anxious life.

By deciding every day to deal with your relationships, your personal environment, your health and healing, and your mindset and emotions . . .

You can quit running.

Stop fighting.

Stop hiding.

You can acknowledge the alarms.

Identify their origin.

And, believe it or not, turn and stare down anxious threats with the assurance that you're capable of responding in ways that will deliver a new kind of life for you, your family, your community, and beyond.

We're talking about changing your family tree.

We're aiming for a life that faces and accepts the pain and heartbreaks and grief, and yet finds joy and community and possibility and hope . . . regardless of what comes next.

Are you in?

Let's go.

CHAPTER 1

WE DIDN'T START THE FIRE . . . SORTA

I pulled up the driveway and into my cluttered garage. I hit the button clipped onto my car's visor and waited for the garage door to go down. After a few minutes the small, single light bulb clicked off. My hands were still on the steering wheel when I realized I was sitting in total darkness.

I took a deep breath but didn't make a move to get out of the car. *Not yet.* It felt like there was some kind of band around the bottom of my lungs. I couldn't catch my breath.

Pulling out my phone, I began scrolling through the news sites. It was all terrible, catastrophic news.

My heart started beating faster. I was sitting in silence.

I swiped off the internet and checked my email. I'd just looked at it before I left the office no more than 15 minutes ago. But I checked again anyway. Out of habit. Surprisingly, I had several new messages, and one subject line caught my attention. The email marked "re: Budget Meeting."

My stomach dropped with a warm, heavy feeling. My body felt like someone was standing in the corner of my dark garage with an axe.

I knew no one was trying to kill me. I even muttered to myself, "There's *no one with an axe* . . . chill out!" Still, I took a few more deep breaths before getting out of the car.

Wading through my mess in the garage, I opened the door to find my wife at the kitchen table. I immediately launched into a play-by-play of my day, letting her know who the idiots were at work, who didn't know what they were doing, and who was cheating on their wife. Most importantly, I gave her my latest diatribe on some new *research*[7] about a diet that would help me focus better, lose weight, make me a better man . . . and oh yeah, I wanted to plant a huge garden in our postage-stamp backyard in case we have a global food shortage.

My wife tried hard to stay tuned in, but I wasn't easy to follow.

She asked if I'd sent in the student loan payments and paid the credit card bills. I thought for a minute. I didn't remember, so I made something up. *"Yes" on the credit card, I think; "no" on one of the student loans. I'd check on that later.*

After dinner, I was watching television and mindlessly

---

[7] And to be clear, by *research*, I mean some internet article I'd stumbled across, some forwarded email I'd received, or some conversation I'd overheard in line for coffee. I was looking for anyone, anywhere who would confirm what I wanted to be true. It was ridiculous.

scrolling the internet. I ended up buying some shoes on one of our credit cards. As soon as I saw the confirmation for my purchase, a burst of energy bolted through my body. It felt good, as though these shoes would solve something. Then I had the thought to check our credit card balance.

Uh-oh. We were $50 away from the max limit.

Cue the shame. It washed over me and through me.

We owed so much money. Several hundred thousand dollars.

I hated owing people money. Student loans and credit cards and our mortgage and my used truck—it was too much. But money woes weren't the only problem.

Anywhere I looked, I wasn't finding much to feel good about. I was gaining weight, I didn't have any friends around other than the folks I worked with, and I moaned and complained about everything. At work, I constantly whined about feeling undervalued and was convinced I was WAY better at my job than my colleagues who had better titles and made higher salaries.

At about 11:15 p.m., I took my prescription sleep meds and finally faded into the blackhole unconsciousness of chemically induced sleep.

No! No! No! No! No! No!

My eyes flung open and I was instantly awake, my heart pounding like a jackhammer. My painfully exhausted body was slow to move, adding to the panic in my mind. Somewhere deep in my brain, my amygdala was trying to keep me alert. DANGER!

I fumbled around on the floor for my phone to see what time it was. I had a pile of books, some clothes, and a few biohacker gadgets on my side of the bed, and I kept knocking things around until I finally grabbed hold of my phone.

1:37 a.m.

I just stared at the glowing numbers.

I would have sworn it was 6 a.m.

Not even close.

"Come *on!*" I hissed, trying not to wake my wife. "It's every night!"

Moving the mess out of the way, I crawled out of bed and went to the living room. I knew I was done sleeping for the night and wanted to make good use of the time.

I sat down on the couch and covered up with my new weighted anxiety blanket. I re-opened my laptop and headed back to the news sites, clicking and scrolling on more doom and gloom. I answered a mad rush of work emails and then played some games on my phone until lightly dozing off sometime around 3:30.

When the alarm on my phone went off, I felt like I was being pulled from underwater. It was 5:30 a.m. Like a good soldier, I got up, stumbled out of the house, and drove to the gym. 'Cause that's what I was supposed to do.

This wasn't just some random, no good, very bad day.

This was every day.

This was the life I had created.

For the most part, I was really trying to do what I was being told to do. The loans, the jobs, the house, the cars, the sleep meds, the politics and "Don't miss a second of the news . . ."

And it was destroying me and those I loved.

So imagine my surprise when, more than a decade later, I found out: This isn't just my life. This is almost everyone's life.

In some version of anxiety or another, millions of you aren't sleeping, you're drowning in debt, being hammered by trauma and pain, feeling lonely or insecure, and you have no boundaries.

We live anxious lives, and it is destroying us.

HOW WE GOT HERE

For the past two decades I have talked with, counseled, coached, or walked alongside people from every walk of life.

Parents whose kids have not lived up to their expectations.

Kids who are responsible for making sure Dad doesn't get angry or Mom doesn't feel lonely.

Grieving widows who are trying to rebuild their lives out of ash.

I've looked parents in the eye and told them their child is no longer alive.

I've watched folks crumble in the aftermath of abuse, losing their job, or finding out their spouse has cheated.

I've spoken at or attended more memorial services than I can remember.

I've sat with folks who don't have enough money to

eat and have no one to call. People who've been sexually assaulted and abused. People who have been kicked and stomped to the margins for not looking or living like everyone else.

I have also spent countless hours with people whose lives aren't yet in ashes but the fires are burning and they can't breathe through the smoke.

People up to their eyeballs in debt who, after clarinet lessons, travel soccer, the school dance recital, and yet another tuition increase, find themselves with no margin.

People doing more work for less money with barely enough to make it through the month. Worried because the air conditioner is on life support, milk is a thousand dollars a gallon, and eggs are trading on Wall Street.

As I look deeply in my own mirror, this is me and my family too.

You and me and all of us.

We have created frantic, chaotic, roller-coaster lives.

We've either been dropped into anxious ecosystems or we've built our own anxious lives from the ground up. And somewhere along the way, we became convinced this was freedom. Or, we know there's more to life but we don't know where to turn.

We're anxious on the way to work. Anxious on the way home from work.

We are glued to our phones for the latest housing and stock market numbers. If one card falls, the whole house of cards comes crashing down.

We've outsourced romance to *The Bachelor*, our homes to Chip and Joanna, our spiritual lives to Instagram and the scientific method, and our kids to digital babysitters.

We snap at our children, look to remove stress by adding things (a new day planner, yoga class, or fad diet), use chemicals to wake up in the morning, and rely on pills and drinks to drag ourselves into the dark waters of sleep at night.

All the while, we're living in an environment we were never made for.

Let me say that again another way, because it's the main premise of this book: **We've created a world our bodies cannot exist in.**

Every day in a thousand ways, our bodies are screaming at us, sounding the alarms that we're disconnected and lonely. We're unsafe and unhealthy. We've given away all our autonomy, and now bosses and mortgage companies and in-laws and academic advisors are controlling our lives.

And then it happens.

You're meeting someone at a hotel who's not your wife.

You're pouring vodka into your coffee mug first thing in the morning.

You're padding your hours on your timecard.

Or you're yelling at your kids or disappearing from your spouse into a cavern of silence like an angry bear.

You stop going to church.

You and your husband stop having sex. You and your wife have no common purpose—you're just glorified roommates, each living your own life in parallel.

You quit your job and then beg to get it back. Three weeks in and you're already back on LinkedIn, looking for other leads.

You sell your home, buy something that's more "you," and lock yourself into a mortgage you'll never pay off.

Does any of this sound familiar?

We don't know how we got here, what we're doing, or where to go from here. But we know *anxious, worried,* and *paralyzed by fear*.

WITHOUT BOUNDARIES

The first thing to go is our boundaries. We quit critically thinking for ourselves and outsource our thoughts and feelings to others who don't have our best interests at heart.

We let politicians and organizations tell us who to hate. We let social media focus us on how much we lack. We let our parents decide where we'll spend the holidays and our kids dictate what we eat. We let advertisers prescribe how to spend our money and schools assess what's wrong with our kids.

And over time, all these voices become our voice.

We say to our younger self—the one with the dreams, and hopes, and the radical imagination—"Shut your mouth and go back to your room." Then we walk into the next busy, anesthetizing thing with no intentionality, no plan, and no idea why.

We listen to untrained, uninformed, or unwise voices, and we follow them willingly into the next distraction. The latest money hack or get-rich scheme. The next "money-back guaranteed" exercise program. An internet romance. A new house or car. A must-see Netflix series.

Numbed.

We are fried, exhausted, and burned out.

OF COURSE there's a massive rise in anxiety in our homes, our lives, and our world!

THE QUESTION OF ANXIETY

The longer I sit with hurting people and study the ins and outs of anxiety (or most other mental-health diagnostics, for that matter), the more I'm convinced that there are few, if any, crazy people.

Please hear me.

I don't think you're crazy.

I don't think you're broken down like an old, rusty bicycle.

And neither is your one cousin who's always asking you for money, the girl from high school who's in jail, or the guy who installed that way-loud "muffler" on his sports car.

I believe people are just trying to find ways to hurt less, be heard and seen, find safety, connect with others, and survive.

And they'll do whatever it takes.

I'm doing whatever it takes.

When folks ask me questions about anxiety, they are rarely asking me diagnostic or clinical questions. They are asking:

"What is wrong with my body?"

"Do I have a disease?"

"Will I have to take meds forever?"

"Is my kid normal?"

"Is my marriage done for good?"

"Can I ever be comfortable in a room full of people?"

"Do I have a chance at losing the weight?"

"Will the bullying ever stop?"

They're asking if they'll always be scared of disappointing their father, or if they'll be able to eat out or ride the subway without being afraid.

They're asking if they can ever hope to love again.

They're desperate to know if they're worth being loved.

And while I honor these questions and have spent years asking them myself, I am now convinced that in most cases, they are the wrong questions.

They are questions about smoke and alarm systems, not about fire and chaotic lives and restoration.

This is why I wrote this book.

DARK, EVEN FOR ME

I've read back over this chapter several times.

It feels like too much. Too many lists. Too much coming at the reader. It's dark, even for me. It doesn't feel like there's much hope.

In the original draft, I tried to start this book with some comic humor and a funny story, but it rang false. The world has lost its mind, and things are not as they could be. I'm not going to run from that truth.

Or from the fact that you and I have constructed a roller coaster and decided to call it home, even though everything is turned upside down.

But I also see hope everywhere.

I need you to trust me on this.

I would not have written this book if I didn't believe there is hope. For you, for me, for our kids, for the people we love, and for our world.

I've heard it in thousands and thousands of people. I've seen it in my friends and neighbors. I've experienced it in my home.

There is light bursting forth.

I believe this with every fiber of my being.

Take a deep breath and imagine with me for a moment.

You wake in the morning.

You sit up and you take a few full breaths. Your sleep was deep and restorative, like usual. You get out of bed and, instead of a death-sprint to the espresso machine, you take a long walk outside or knock out a brutal workout at your local gym. And *then* you grab a coffee, not because you have to but because you want to. Or you laugh at the chaos of getting the kids ready for school, and you and your young son have to change shirts because a water fight got playfully out of hand.

You check your bank balance and you have a cash emergency fund. You owe no one anything except for your mortgage—or maybe not even that. And though you're disappointed to be leaving your job over a narcissistic boss, you're not terrified or worried. You've got six months of savings, and career options, and deeply held values about your own self-worth.

You've made peace with your body—you don't believe you're ugly or disgusting anymore. Or that you're not enough. Or that no one will ever love you. You believe you're worth taking care of. And you believe in consistency and discipline over endless fads and hacks.

And you don't hate. As the Avett Brothers sing, you have "no hard feelings." You love and give recklessly. You let people over in traffic, you assume the best, and you choose your few fights wisely.

You do snap at your wife and raise your voice at your kids. But you immediately stop everything, get at eye level, and deeply apologize, asking what you can do to restore the relationship.

You weep openly with friends at the passing of your dad.

You set boundaries for the holidays, and you feel super-guilty but not resentful.

You march in the streets when you need to march. You scroll past social media comments without commenting. You experience change as an opportunity, not something to run from.

You have hard conversations with a counselor or your group of friends who religiously meet every week.

You leave your town when it's time for a new thing, even though it's all you've known.

You are resilient, disciplined, and courageous. And kind, joyful, peaceful, and patient.

This, my friends, is a non-anxious life.

THE STRATEGY

You'll get tired of me saying this, but I'm going to keep repeating it: **Anxiety is not the problem.**

The problem is that we are unsafe, disconnected, unhealthy, and living like we have no say in what happens next.

In this book, I'm going to give you a strategy for something better than just muffling the anxiety alarms. This is the way to build a non-anxious life.

Make no mistake, I didn't invent this approach. It's not some vision-board manifestation or some cute social media conglomeration. This path is informed by ancient wisdom, neuroscience, psychology and physiology, real-world application, and personal experiences.

As I said in the introduction, this path has been traversed over centuries.

We need to know the way because life is hard. Really hard. It will keep throwing punches, and elbows, and kicks. You'll get fired and lose loved ones and hurt those you care about. But we can no longer try to avoid these bad things. We must build a resilient, non-anxious life that allows us to absorb the hits.

And every single one of us will get hit. A lot.

The death rate on this quest called life is 100 percent. None of us gets out of this adventure alive.

Nevertheless, I want to continually pull our focus away

from an obsession with fixing our anxious bodies, minds, and lives, or healing from acute anxiety (or even some hyper-specific diagnosis), and instead focus on the lives we have created that keep setting off our body's innate alarm systems.

Let's worry less about the alarms and focus more on what's causing them to sound off in the first place.

Starting with the next chapter, I want to transform everything you think you know about anxiety—changing the way you see it, understand it, and in some cases, even experience it. In chapter 2, we will take a deep dive into what anxiety is, what it isn't, and how we have all ended up so anxious and spun out. If you ever read *Redefining Anxiety*, some of this might be familiar to you, but don't skip over it. It will be important for us all to be on the same page as we head onto the path.

Let's redefine anxiety.

CHAPTER 2

REDEFINING ANXIETY

In 2008, President George W. Bush gave an address warning about the coming economic meltdown.[8] At the time, I was oblivious to any sort of happenings with the stock market or the greater economy.[9] I didn't have any money, so naturally I thought, *That economic stuff doesn't matter to me.*

I was woefully mistaken.

My wife and I were renting a small house from the university where we both worked. We owed six figures in student loan debt, and I was lavishly adding to it to fund yet another graduate degree. We were in a new town with new

---

[8] This was back when people trusted presidents and press conferences were actual events. This may sound hard to believe, but Americans used to either agree or disagree with politicians while generally trusting that our leaders had the best intentions in mind for the country. A presidential press conference was a stop-what-you're-doing moment.

[9] I was oblivious to pretty much everything. My wife assures me I still am.

jobs and new colleagues. In the midst of collecting data for a dissertation, I was hopping from one fad diet to another, working 70 hours a week, and I didn't think twice about forgoing "luxuries" like sleep and community.

I was trying to crush it and kill it and do all things bro-wisdom. And I was both exhausted and exhausting to be around.

I was walking through the living room when the television cut away from our regularly scheduled program to a live-feed of a grim President Bush at the podium. I remember standing in front of the TV, frozen, as the President of the United States told us that our nation was perilously close to a financial implosion. He noted how we were all feeling anxiety.

And I remember how my heart stopped beating in an orderly fashion.

I actually felt it.

The president kept talking, and his words soon became Charlie Brown teacher-speak.

My body went fully limbic. Thoughts and worries spun up automatically, turning my mind into a blender. Something called "mortgage-backed securities" were threatening to send us back to the Stone Age, and there was nothing any of us ordinary citizens could do about it. My body was paralyzed by the idea that some nameless, faceless people could make crooked deals in the back room of some banking institution and ruin families and businesses and the country. Or that short-minded incentives, spread across multiple sectors of an industry, could cave in on themselves and cost people everything.

In fact, as I type this, my heart is speeding up again. My body still remembers.

But this isn't where the story began.

Let's back up a few decades.

Back to my childhood home. A home filled with love, community service, faith, and angst. Loads of angst.

Angst because we didn't have money. We were always struggling financially.

My dad was a police officer, and my community didn't think enough of police officers to pay them a decent wage. We did without a lot of things and put other things on credit cards. My parents shared a single used station wagon, and we lived in a modest home. Though we didn't miss a meal and we always had shoes, I know people from our church quietly helped. Generous folks would give us excellent hand-me-down clothes and buy us meals, and one year, people broke into our house and piled Christmas gifts under our tree.

Ever since I could remember, I hated money. Not really money itself, but the stress it caused within our home. I hated the things we couldn't afford. I hated the way a lack of money unfairly seemed to signal to the community that my family was somehow less-than. I hated the way I would spend my mowing money the second I got it in a scarcity-fueled mania.

Money became synonymous with shame and scarcity.

As I grew older, I hated the charges and fees and anxiety that went along with credit cards. Yet I upped the ante of money stress with my own idiotic, self-sabotaging choices. I was reckless with borrowing and spending. I dug myself a massive financial hole trying to keep up with appearances and enjoy the comforts I felt I missed out on as a kid. I attempted to solve my childhood stress of not having enough with the adult stress of owing money on credit cards, car notes, and student loans.

Years later, as I watched the president's address, these beliefs and feelings resurfaced in the living room of our tiny rental home.

I was in full fight-or-flight as soon as I heard his words. I'm not exaggerating. I ended up in the hospital some months later. My body was running, fighting, and hiding—desperately trying to do something about something I couldn't do anything about—and I was chaotic, not-sleeping, way-overeating, out-of-my-mind stressed and angry.

My body was trying to let me know I wasn't safe. That I was alone. That I had outsourced the greater decisions being made about my future.

This was anxiety.

SO WHAT IS ANXIETY?

Before we *redefine* anxiety, we have to first explore how medical providers, mental-health practitioners, and insurance companies are taught to define it. So alas, we must explore the DSM-5.

Controversially known as the "psychiatric bible," the fifth

edition of the *Diagnostic and Statistical Manual of Mental Disorders* (DSM-5) suggests "anxiety disorders . . . share features of excessive fear and anxiety and related behavioral disturbances." The manual goes on to state that "anxiety disorders differ from one another in the types of objects or situations that induce fear, anxiety, or avoidance behavior, and the associated cognitive ideation."[10]

If you think this isn't clear, put on your nerd hat, because it gets worse.

The DSM-5 breaks down anxiety disorders into different types, such as separation anxiety, selective mutism, phobias, social anxiety, and more. It places stress-related disorders (like post-traumatic stress), disordered eating, obsessive-compulsive disorders, and many other anxiety- and stress-based challenges into entirely separate diagnostic categories even though there is significant overlap in symptoms, stressors, and responses. This often results in diagnostic *co-morbidity*, meaning that a person is diagnosed with multiple psychological disorders at the same time.

If you're anything like me, you find this less than helpful.

Personally, I don't care for the DSM's overly sophisticated slicing-and-dicing of the human experience. It's like we spilled milk on the floor and we are all standing around arguing about it, talking about it, naming different types of

---

[10] American Psychiatric Association, *Diagnostic and Statistical Manual of Mental Disorders, Fifth Edition, Text Revision (DSM-5-TR)* (Washington, DC: APA Publishing, 2022), 189.

spills, trying to come up with theories on spills and the history of spills . . . and no one is cleaning up the milk.

What are we doing?

And before my fellow mental-health professionals start throwing rocks, I do believe the diagnostic manual(s) have a role to play. They help the professionals talk to one another in a common language, they allow researchers to stay consistent in and across research studies, and they make it easier for insurance companies to pay mental-health providers for their services.[11] For the professionals, the codifications and charts and graphs might prove helpful in certain applications. And yes, a diagnosis can be useful for someone who is hurting. It names the dragon and puts a label on a person's challenges. Under the care of a trained professional, it can provide direction for treatment. But on the whole, I don't like these labels for several reasons.

First, they often don't represent the human experience. Our body's response to grief, stress, childhood traumas, job loss, relationship challenges, and rumors of war cannot be captured in a series of neat categories and codes. Second, I continue to see diagnostics become identities (we'll discuss this in more detail in chapter 3). People internalize their

---

[11] Most of the time, though admittedly not always, I have about as much use for the DSM as I do for a sudden bout of diarrhea on a dance floor. Apart from its professional purposes, having a copy of the DSM serves as a decent hedge against any of the rest of us ever running out of toilet paper.

diagnostic label(s) and say things like, "I have anxiety," and it becomes a fixed characteristic in their hearts and minds. In time, this identity often becomes the lens through which they see themselves as broken or dysfunctional. Finally, individuals diagnosed with mental-health disorders may have to report diagnostics on certain insurance applications, some professional applications, and in other places. When dealing with real people living real lives, the ends often don't justify the means.

I have friends and colleagues who arc back and forth on this issue—and that's fine. What's not fine is this: turning the body's responses to the challenges of life into a series of clinical categories. This has not helped us curb, heal, or even make a dent in the numbers. In fact, over the past decade, anxiety has escalated. On a rocket ship.

The manuals are not helping.

We have more "understanding" than ever before, yet collectively we're more anxious and burned out than we've ever been. Our homes, our bodies, our kids, our workplaces, our public spaces are anxious, anxious, anxious.

It's time to reimagine our answers to the problem.

REIMAGINING OUR ANSWERS

Let's do a thought-experiment.

Imagine you're sitting on the couch, watching re-runs of *Seinfeld*. Or *Yellowstone* if you prefer your soap operas to be outdoors.

You're procrastinating on a huge project at work, you have a class assignment due for the leadership certificate you're working toward, and several loads of laundry are piled in the corner.

You've silenced a call from your mom three or four times, and your husband (who's still wearing cargo shorts even though the fashion police have clearly called an end to this entire look)[12] is giving you the grumpy, stay-away-from-me, Sunday-Dad vibes.

The whole scene is *blah*. Especially the shorts.

Suddenly, out of nowhere, the kitchen smoke alarm goes off. It's so loud—like someone parked an ambulance right behind your couch and turned up the sirens.

At first, you just try to ignore it. Soon, you grab your couch cushions and make a sandwich with your face, trying to block the sound. It's still too loud.

You notice your cell phone buzzing and *it's your mom. Again.* You reach over and silence the call. Again.

You turn up the volume on the television as loud as it will go.

The alarm is pulsing. Piercing.

Your head starts pounding and now your stomach is hurting. *It just won't stop.*

You have another idea.

---

[12] I will never—never!—give up my cargo shorts. Who knows when I might need to go on an archaeological dig or Limp Bizkit might need me to play guitar for their comeback tour?

Grabbing a roll of duct tape and a few pillows off the couch, you climb up on a chair in the kitchen and tightly duct tape the pillows around the alarm.

This makes a big difference. You congratulate yourself, climb down, put the chair back, and return to the living room to watch your show. The alarm is still loud, but not like it was.

Though there's smoke everywhere, and you can hardly breathe, you can still make out your television. You return to where you were sitting and focus on the wisps of light breaking through the haze.

CRASH!

The back room of your house collapses. Smoke is everywhere. The alarms up and down the back hallway begin screeching, one after another.

You instinctively grab a chair and head for the nearest alarm. You jam in a screwdriver, pop off the battery cover, and rip out the batteries. The alarm goes silent. You take off running down the hall, hustling from room to room, prying the batteries out of each little plastic disc.

Ahhhh. The alarms are quiet except for the one in the kitchen, but you can put up with that one thanks to the pillows and duct tape.

You sit back down on the couch, barely able to breathe from the billowing smoke, but thrilled that you finally shut up the alarms. Making yourself a drink, you throw your feet up on the coffee table, wave the smoke away from your immediate area, and continue watching the show.

Suddenly, the ceiling caves in over the dining room table. Sheetrock and insulation and the light fixture come crashing down, ripping the pillows off the alarm. The ceiling is roiling with flames, and now the cabinets are on fire too.

You're in a swirl of noise, fire, flames, and smoke. You can't see anything, and you can't fully inhale. Everything is on fire.

You try to enjoy the last few moments . . .

As your home burns down around you.

This is me and this is you.

This is our schools and our political parties, our churches and our families.

This is anxiety.

So what is anxiety?

Hang on to your hats, ladies and gentlemen. *Drumroll, please.*

Anxiety is simply an alarm.

That's it.

I'm not being flippant or disrespectful. I've seen doctors and specialists and taken medication for my own debilitating anxiety. I have two PhDs and have taught graduate counseling courses. I've also walked alongside countless anxious, stressed, and burned-out individuals. I know anxiety personally, intellectually, and professionally.

Anxiety is just an alarm.

In the thought-experiment above, you were running around, trying to chase down the alarms while your home burned to the ground. You ignored the smoke, the flames, and the phone calls from a loved one. You were single-mindedly obsessed with turning off the alarms.

And it almost cost you everything.

The Alarms

The anxiety alarms generally begin sounding for one or more of the following four reasons:

1. Your body senses you are alone and disconnected from your friends, family, community, or tribe. You are lonely and on your own.
2. Your body senses you are unsafe, or a place, a person, or a group of people is unsafe.
3. Your body recognizes it is unhealthy, overstimulated, sleep-deprived, or struggling with relational and physical boundaries, trauma, illness, drug-use, hormone dysregulation, or other health or healing concerns.
4. Your body understands you don't have autonomy in your life (due to a relationship or your environment, for example). Someone or something else is making decisions about how you will live your life.

Consider this: Anxiety is generally your body's way of trying to take care of you and get your attention. Through the right lens, anxiety can even be considered a friend.

Dr. Wendy Suzuki, who is a professor of neural science and psychology at New York University, calls anxiety "good."[13] A loud, annoying, and at times brutally relentless friend for sure, but a good friend nonetheless. Anxiety is just trying to keep you alive, and safe, and out of harm's way.

Dr. Suzuki further says anxiety is our "psychological and physical response to stress. . . . Anxiety is a hardwired threat response that our brain-body uses to protect us."[14] It's the instinctive call to get up and run or to stand and fight against some imagined future enemy or calamity— emphasis on *future*.

The great Stanford researcher and professor Robert Sapolsky describes anxiety this way: "Anxiety is about the dread and foreboding and your imagination running away with you. . . . It is where constant vigilance is the only hope of effectively protecting yourself."[15] In other words, anxiety is the alarm spinning up feelings and stories against any future danger that might come at you. Anxiety calls you to prepare for war.

So yes, anxiety is simply an alarm.

But the alarms are loud. Anxiety is grueling, powerful, and debilitating. Frustratingly, while one part of your brain

---

[13] Wendy Suzuki, *Good Anxiety: Harnessing the Power of the Most Misunderstood Emotion* (New York: Atria Books, 2021), 5.
[14] Suzuki, *Good Anxiety*, 13, 16.
[15] Robert M. Sapolsky, *Why Zebras Don't Get Ulcers* (New York: St. Martin's Press, 2004), 319.

and body is busy sounding the alarms, another part of your brain and body kicks into action to quiet them down. This creates a habit loop, and the anxiety alarms become automated. *Ugh.*

Habits and Addictions

After writing *Redefining Anxiety*, I was introduced to the work of Dr. Jud Brewer, Director of Research and Innovation at Brown University's Mindfulness Center and a professor at Brown Medical School. He is an expert's expert who has done extensive research on anxiety, mindfulness, and behavior transformation. Dr. Brewer suggests that anxiety, the alarm system residing deep in your brain, is a "reward-based learning system"[16] elegant in its simplicity yet extraordinary in its effectiveness. Thus anxiety can become a habit.

Don't miss how profound this is. Your alarms, according to Dr. Brewer, turn into a feedback loop of "trigger – behavior – reward."[17] Before long, anxiety can become your default setting. Here's an example:

> My body is triggered by some event—let's say in my case, something about money. It sets off my anxiety alarms and sends my body into fight, flight, or freeze.

---

[16] Judson Brewer, *Unwinding Anxiety: Train Your Brain to Heal Your Mind* (New York: Avery, Penguin Random House, 2021), 31.
[17] Brewer, *Unwinding Anxiety*, 33.

In response, maybe I shut off the media with the bad financial report to avoid the information altogether. Or maybe I'm filled with anger and I take it out on some unsuspecting delivery driver. Or maybe I grab a drink and another drink, or a bag of candy. Or I buy something just because. Or I scroll myself into comfortable numbness.

For a moment, my body feels good. The alarms are quiet. I get the feeling of superiority. The sugar rush. The shopper's high. My brain craves the reward of being numb or powerful or satisfied, and the feedback loop has been created.

Brewer says we can become addicted to "shopping . . . , pining away for that special someone . . . , computer gaming . . . , continued eating . . . , daydreaming . . . , social media checking . . . , worrying,"[18] and more. Anything that becomes a distraction or a pacifier from the source of anxiety (the fires) can, over time, become an addiction.

Best-selling author James Clear says, "Habits are the small decisions you make and actions you perform every day."[19] For most habitual actions, what you're doing has been automated—you act without thinking. Like grabbing some coffee every time you leave the house. Like yelling when you're mad, exercising as soon as you wake up, or grabbing a cookie anytime you walk by the jar. An addiction, on the

---

[18] Brewer, *Unwinding Anxiety*, 29.
[19] James Clear, *Atomic Habits* (New York: Avery, 2018), 6.

other hand, is a compulsive action you continue to do even when it's clear the action is harmful.

What Dr. Brewer so beautifully articulates is that at first, anxiety is simply an alarm that sounds in response to a trigger. Over time, the actions that turn down the alarms become habits. We reach for our phone, a doughnut, or a drink whenever we get stressed. Eventually, these habits develop into full-blown addictions.

We become addicted to the alarms.

There is some debate in the scientific community that we can even become addicted to the stress chemicals like cortisol and adrenaline that make us feel pumped up and ready to take on the world.[20] Or that we can get hooked on the depressing chemicals that keep us low and hidden.

-----

[20] There appears to be some disagreement in the literature as to whether addictions are actually habits, diseases, or learned behaviors—or some of all three. It could be that our bodies get physically addicted to the stress hormones released during the fight-or-flight cycle. Or it could be that we have a psychological addiction to the feeling of power we get from cortisol and adrenaline pulsing through our veins. Or it might be that our body is addicted to the alcohol or heroin or pornography or rage, and it can get us to partake in those behaviors by spinning up the anxiety alarms at the slightest impulse.

My reading of the literature is that it's probably a concoction of all three of these theories, though in the day to day it doesn't matter much. It's just important to understand that our bodies can become addicted to anxiety—the entire habit loop. From the alarms, to actions, to the rewards.

Dr. Brewer says it this way: "A thought or emotion triggers your brain to start worrying. This results in avoiding the negative thought or emotion, which feels more rewarding than the original thought or emotion."[21]

Your body needs a drink or a pat on the back? Sound the alarm.

Your body needs a hit of fight-or-flight chemicals like cortisol or adrenaline? Pick a fight with your spouse or boss and let your internal chemistry do its work.

Everything quickly becomes chaos.

We get so busy avoiding alarms, creating alternative routes to the same places, and struggling in our addictions, that we miss the big picture. And here's one more frustrating twist: if our brain is addicted to the alarms, but there are no death traps in sight, it may spin up a painful story from the past, or choose to interpret current inputs in a tragically negative way—news reports, social media posts, or those email forwards from your mom that look a lot like end-times conspiracy theories, but she calls them "facts."

Your mind will begin to see dragons and demons and bogeymen everywhere in order to satisfy the alarm addiction. And whether it's cortisol or a new girlfriend or that extra beer, it will get what it wants.

As we try to avoid them, the anxiety alarms will grow stronger and louder.

---

[21] Brewer, *Unwinding Anxiety*, 34.

MEMORY, ACTION, AND GRIEF

Anxiety alarms are connected to the parts of our brain that filter and direct memories and emotions. When we experience bad things or scary things or dangerous things, our body puts a GPS pin over that person, object, or experience. This happens with major acute traumas, and it also happens in rather routine moments across a person's life.

Your anxiety alarms are intent on survival. They don't care if you're happy. They don't care if you're living your best life. Their job is to keep you safe. And they'll resurface throughout your life, in seemingly unconnected moments.

If a drunk driver hit your car from the passenger side when you were a kid, your body may always flinch, avert, or become alerted every time a car is headed your way from that side. Your brain remembers the time you got hurt, and it's determined to never get hurt like that again.

This sort of hyper-vigilant flinching might be fine when you're driving a car, but it can cause havoc in your relationships.

Maybe you learned at a young age that it was best for you to disappear when you heard Dad's truck rumbling up the driveway. Or maybe it was your job to distract Mom after she'd been drinking so that she wouldn't hit your little brother. And now you're an adult, with children of your own, and you find your heart rate accelerating every time you hear your garage door open. Or when your wife gets frustrated with your son. Your body switches to autopilot, seeking to hide or reaching for something soothing. Or without warning, your body prepares for war, because it remembers, and you find yourself lacing up your gloves, ready to fight.

Across our lives, in situations like these and so many more, we have remembered—and experienced—anxiety. Anxiety is connected to memory.

From Memory to Action

Your body remembers the loud BANGS from your first deployment. It remembers the pain and the blood and the tears. In an effort to protect you, your body attaches anxiety alarms to loud noises and unexpected movements. It goes off when your wife drops something in the kitchen. Or when someone comes running up to you at the curb outside of Costco to sell you Girl Scout cookies.

Your body remembers what it was like to be fired. Or assaulted. Or left to raise the kids alone after the wreck. Or what you saw at the movies and on the news. It's making notes, opening new files on new threats, and always scanning the environment for more threats. Your body is constantly dropping pins.

It knows just how desperate and scary your financial situation is. It knows poverty. Getting made fun of. Homelessness. Or being cheated on.

Your body remembers and sounds the alarms over and over and over again.

Every time the boss calls an emergency meeting.

Every time a man raises his voice.

Every time your local weather station issues a "red alert."

The alarms go off, and your alarm system can't tell the difference between the past or present or future. It struggles to decipher between your imagination and real life. If your system had a motto, it would be: *Better safe than sorry.* Better to sound the alarm and be safe, than to be in danger and remain quiet.[22]

Being wrong in the first situation is annoying and embarrassing. Get it wrong in the second one and you may not get out alive. So better to sound the alarms, just in case.

After a while, we'll do anything to numb out or distract ourselves from the piercing shrill.

- Food
- Drugs
- Alcohol
- Work
- Googling "what happened to the cast of Dawson's Creek" with a work deadline looming
- Rage and anger
- Imaginary conversations and obsessive thinking

---

[22] They may also sound every time your husband heads out in public wearing black socks, Crocs, and shorts. Or when your wife exclaims how happy she is that mom jeans are *finally* back in style.

- Sex
- Exercise
- Trying to be perfect
- Being right and power plays
- Starting fights
- Buying and buying and buying (even when you can't afford it)
- Collecting and organizing and hoarding stuff
- Cleaning the house
- Mercilessly talking down to ourselves
- Doom-scrolling social media
- Staying up-to-the-minute on every current news headline, global tragedy, or climate concern
- More data and more data and more data

Many of these responses are good in the right context. Great, even. But when used to deflect, avoid, or cover up, they become habits. And then addictions. And then identities. Powerful devices to keep the real world at bay. In short order, anxiety can become a miserable, stressful, unpeaceful way of avoidantly navigating the world.

These numbing devices usually work for a while. Some of them work really well. They can quiet the alarms and provide temporary relief. But the fire of your life will rage on and on. And when we try to cover up or just squash the alarms, we also shut off the good things too. As Dr. Brené Brown, research professor and best-selling author, reminds us: joy and pain are on the same switch. So when the batteries are removed, the whole system shuts down. We say goodbye to both the scary things and the good things.

And we'll often do anything to keep avoiding. Our memories light us up and enact our minds and bodies, and we run off trying to control the variables through external action or through rumination and looping thoughts.

Excessive Action (aka, Solving for Toilet Paper)

Dr. Rollo May, one of the great fathers of modern psychotherapy, suggests that "one means of allaying anxiety is frantic activity."[23] He further asserts that powerlessness in the face of potential destruction, combined with our cultural ethos that *with hard work we can do anything*, leads to an excessive form of activism.

Translated: we become human hurricanes.

Without realizing it, we find ourselves going and going and running and striving. We're fighting everyone. Or running from everything. Or filling up our calendars as a way to prove our worth. Or we're eating everything in sight, drinking so much, watching too much news, or constantly finding someone new to sleep with.

In a rush to *do something now*, anxiety pushes us to Costco so we can buy the remaining toilet paper, tubs of almond butter, and AA batteries before anyone else figures out *it's all*

---

[23] Rollo May, *The Meaning of Anxiety* (New York: W. W. Norton & Company, 2015 reissue), 40.

coming down! We'll be able to wipe with comfortable triple-ply as the zombies smash out our windows.

Remember the run on toilet paper during the Covid shutdown? This was individual and collective anxiety played out like a Farrelly Brothers movie. When we were faced with the ugly truth that we were in control of almost nothing in our lives, our bodies began screaming at us to DO SOMETHING! The anxiety alarms were ringing! So what did we do?

We bought lots and lots of toilet paper. More accurately, we bought all of it. Until the shelves were empty.

Did Covid cause massive, explosive diarrhea? Nope.

But we stocked up on toilet paper anyway. And for one brief moment, our bodies felt at peace. Our dopamine and serotonin high-fived the norepinephrine and the cortisol and jointly declared, "We can't control much, but we can wipe our butts with luxury!"

It was one of those times in life we can all look back on with some collective silly-guilt and shake our heads.

But the impulse to do something can take on a much more serious role. As we discussed earlier, your body puts a GPS pin on pain, hurt, and things that can get you killed. Things it's seen (or imagined) before. It remembers when your friend died, when your long-term girlfriend cheated, or when your adult kid stole from you for the fifth time. The alarms push you to send a hundred desperate text messages in an hour, or to believe *I can never love and trust again*, or to obsess over who's to blame and exactly how. Just do something!

Action without Moving a Muscle

Often, we attempt to activate ourselves, not with physical action but *with our thoughts*. We try to pre-plan, rehearse, perfect, and otherwise come up with every possible answer to every limitless possibility we can imagine. We smash the gas pedal to the floor without putting the car in drive. And even though we're only catastrophizing the end of the world in our minds, or we're only being meticulous in our dreams, our bodies are responding as though these scenarios are happening in the real world.

These types of internal actions are called rumination (or excessive worry) and perfectionism.

Rumination

Have you ever stood in the shower with the hot water running over your shoulders and down your back while having an imaginary conversation with your boss?

You know the one.

The imaginary fight where you say just the right thing, the whole room believes you just won the argument, your boss comes to his senses, begs your forgiveness, and offers you a 20 percent raise and a promotion on the spot—and your colleagues break into wild applause.

Then you get soap in your eyes and snap back to reality.[24]

---

[24] Oh, there goes Rabbit! . . .

Or have you ever been sitting at a traffic light and an image of your deceased father, your hurting child, or your wife's affair lightning-bolts into your mind? I'm talking about specific pictures or images that rattle your bones. And instead of zooming out, you zoom in and replay (or creatively imagine) every aspect of that relationship or situation in high definition?

This is rumination. The spinning and spinning of excessive worry. Our brains are trying to intellectually control things we have absolutely no control over. It's your mind running through game-time scenarios when there's no game being played. And whether it's a real-life disagreement, an imagined moment in time, or simply a rehearsal of potential fights to come, our bodies gear up to fight or run all the same.

Here's what's so annoying: Rumination and anxious thoughts can feel like beneficial activity. Like you're protecting yourself from some future calamity. If you imagine your husband dying in a car wreck enough times, for example, you'll be ready should it ever actually happen.

I promise you won't be.

This is important: **Rumination and worry are a total waste of your time.**

They don't help you think critically, they don't provide you with in-advance answers, and they don't ward off future tragedies through some sort of practice run.

As we'll discuss in the chapters ahead, learning to be mindful of your thoughts (rather than allowing your anxious lightning bolts to become the sum total of your focus) is a powerful practice toward building a non-anxious life.

Perfectionism

Besides showing up as rumination and excessive worry, anxiety can show up as "toxic perfectionism."[25] Best-selling authors Drs. Emily and Amelia Nagoski coined this term to describe the feeling that "if things aren't perfect, they aren't any good." Many of us have been there: believing or behaving like *everything* is ruined if anybody makes one mistake. I've walked off a stage to a standing ovation and had one individual in the book-signing line tell me they didn't like my talk . . . and I didn't sleep that night. I zeroed in on the critic and totally disregarded the thousands of people who loved our time together.

Anytime we are toggling between what's going to happen and how we can make it perfect—or between the curated images on social media and magazine covers—the nagging, prickly shame that accompanies it is actually our body sounding an alarm, informing us that we're a failure. And in those times when we do hit a perfect homerun? The alarms quickly direct us to someone who has already done it before—or better. That person who has made more money, has fewer wrinkles, has a more romantic husband, or is a

---

[25] Emily and Amelia Nagoski, *Burn Out* (New York: Ballantine, 2019), 194–95.

better parent. In this state of mind, our bodies are quick to whisper that we're no good, we've never been good, and we're never going to be good.

And sometimes, when you're conscious enough to avoid manic actions and ruminations, you find yourself quiet and tranquil. It is here that you are honest with yourself about the chasm between what you wanted your life to look like and what it truly looks like in reality.

This is often heartbreaking and sad, its own form of grief.

Grief

I will discuss grief in more detail throughout the book, so I won't spend much time here. But as a quick note, grief is the gap between what you hoped would happen, or how you thought things would be, and what actually happened. When your body detects the gap, it feels your world is not as it should be, so it sounds the alarms.

This could be the result of losing someone or something you loved. Or of feeling that your life was somehow supposed to look different than it does. You thought you'd make more money. Or you'd be more successful. You didn't think your co-worker would throw you under the bus. You thought your dad would live forever or your husband would only have eyes for you. You were certain that little kids don't get cancer or that if you just do the right things, you'd always be blessed.

The alarms can sound when your world explodes and when you're left picking up the pieces.

Grief is accepting reality. Sitting in it. Owning it. No matter how dark and scary reality is.

Make no mistake: Grief is dreadful and uncomfortable. So much so that our bodies try to work around it with actions and movement and overthinking, as I said above. We deny it. We work more hours. We write another grant or paper for publication. We live at the gym—or at the buffet. We play video games until all hours of the night.

But there is no healing without grief. You can't heal without sitting through the alarms and owning your reality. And it's here, in the dark night of your soul, that the small light of hope becomes visible once again.

WHAT IF?

Anxiety is an alarm.

Anxiety can become a habit or an addiction.

Anxiety is trying to keep you safe.

Anxiety can either rage or whisper, demanding we DO SOMETHING to stop it!

But what if we didn't?

Instead of spending dozens of hours searching online for how to heal from anxiety or handle anxiety, or shopping till we drop, or denying our pain, or trying to run faster to get it to stop, what if we didn't throw a blanket over the anxiety in any way?

What if we turned and stared it down?

What if we walked right into the middle of it?

A non-anxious life is one where we pause and listen to what the alarms are telling us.

We head toward the alarms, not away from them.

We'll talk about how to specifically do that very soon. But first, let's recast the narrative around anxiety and talk about what anxiety is not.

CHAPTER 3

WHAT ANXIETY IS NOT (AND A VISION OF SOMETHING DIFFERENT)

L aura exploded into my office.

I was head-down, writing a conduct report. She was wide-eyed and shaking but bravely trying to hold it together.

Laura was one of my favorite graduate students. Brilliant. Strong. Always good for a laugh. I knew then, and time has proven me right: she was going to change the world in so many wonderful ways. But on this day, she was holding a single sheet of paper as though it were used toilet paper.

I invited her to sit down and join me at my conference table. She continued to stand in the doorway.

"I have anxiety!" she exclaimed. "I finally got in at the doctor's office and found out what's wrong with me. Everything I was afraid of came true. What am I supposed to do with this?" She shook the tiny paper angrily. "I have anxiety! I've wasted all this money on grad school, all this time in this stupid town, and now I'm going to be a medicated zombie for the rest of my life!"

She burst into tears and slid down into a nearby chair.

Unfortunately, Laura wasn't the first person to burst into my office, distressed after receiving a diagnostic confirmation. And she wasn't the first person to tell me she believed she was damaged goods. As we talked, and Laura more specifically disclosed her concerns about what she'd been told, I could quickly see that she had taken on a new identity. She was no longer the brilliant, hard-working, hilarious woman who was going to change the world. She "had anxiety." And that was that.

I've lost count of the number of people I've had this conversation with. Laura could have been Paul or Dan or Kelly or Jennifer or others.

When we come to understand that our body is getting our attention by sounding anxiety alarms, it's easy to think we are no longer ourselves. That we have an affliction. A defect.

But we're not broken.

We're not damaged goods.

Our bodies have just finally said, "Things have to change."

THE NARRATIVE

As I said earlier, the narrative we've been given around anxiety is largely nonsense. It's often untrue, unhelpful, and it's burying a generation of people under the faulty idea that they have a disease, or bad genetics, or that they've been cursed and will have to live a life of huddled terror and chronic stress.

If this is you or someone you love, or someone you work with, worship with, or live next to, listen carefully:

Anxiety is not a disease.

I'll say it again for those in the back: Anxiety is not a disease. It's just your body trying to get your attention.

If you're anxious, you are not sick. You may be struggling, but you are not a machine to be fixed or a disease to be cured.[26]

In the introduction to this book, I said that I believe the way we talk about anxiety is wreaking havoc on our culture and our lives. A diagnosis of anxiety is a snapshot, not a feature film. It is a road sign along the highway, not the final destination.

This idea that anxiety is like the flu, and it descends on people, is simply false. If you are struggling with chronic stress, fear, worry, or even full-blown anxiety or panic attacks, it is something you're experiencing, *not who you are*.

If you or someone you love is dealing with anxiety, there is hope and healing and transformation on the other side of the alarms.

In this chapter, I want to reimagine what we know and think and say about anxiety. We've already established that anxiety is an alarm system that can become a habit and, over time, an addiction. We've established what it is, how it works,

---

[26] Obviously, you may be struggling with any number of medical ailments or diseases. But my point here is that anxiety is not a disease. Full stop.

and what it looks like in the wild. But before I move on, I want to clear up some nonsense about anxiety that's out in the public square, especially around two major areas: identity and medication.

First, I want to be clear that anxiety is not an identity. Second, medication is not the only answer for anxiety.

Anxiety Is Not an Identity

In *Redefining Anxiety*, I wrote of my concerns about how the diagnosis of anxiety (or worse, a Google self-diagnosis) becomes an identity for struggling people. A scarlet letter stitched to people's clothing. My concern about diagnostics becoming identity has only grown over the past few years.

As I've previously mentioned, an anxiety diagnosis can help provide direction for treatment and a name for the dragon—the cluster of symptoms you are experiencing or feeling. A diagnosis can also serve to help a person feel not-so-alone. When given a diagnosis, you can become aware of the countless struggling and courageous men and women who are going through the same thing. But it's been my experience and observation that something else is going on.

When someone receives a diagnosis, they are given a name for what is happening in their bodies, and they are also stamped with a label. A label they must then report indefinitely on insurance forms, medical paperwork, and certain employment and educational applications. Similar to when an oncologist tells your dad he has cancer, a clinical mental-health diagnosis sometimes states: You *have* anxiety, or obsessive-compulsive disorder, or post-traumatic stress disorder. You *are* depressed.

The story you're told is: You have it. It's all over you. It fell from the sky or you caught it from the water you drink. You had traumatic experiences as a young child and you're forever damaged. There's no escaping now!

In our current ethos, a diagnosis is now *who you are*. And once you've internalized it, this story surrounding your identity is very, very hard to change. As Dr. Brené Brown says, "Whatever you go looking for, you are sure to find."

When you believe you *have anxiety*, you begin to see signs of it everywhere: In people and situations that make you nervous. In hard conversations. In obstacles at work. In disagreements with your spouse. Over time, anxiety can be a badge, a context for your struggling body, and an excuse—all at the same time.

While reading the manuscript of one of his books, Dr. Jud Brewer's editor remarked, "People romanticize their anxiety and/or stress. They wear it like a badge of honor, without which they would be a lesser person, or worse, lose a sense of purpose. To many, stress equals success. . . . If you are stressed, you are making a contribution. If you're not stressed, you're a loser."[27]

After receiving her diagnosis, Laura went where everybody goes for information: the internet. She internalized the

---

[27] Brewer, *Unwinding Anxiety*, 80.

forecasts about her future. About how she would never be able to hold a job. About how she shouldn't expect to ever enjoy a stable, loving relationship. How she would always be on meds and feel jittery and scattered.

Her life went from one of limitless possibilities to one of determined toil based on a single conversation with an over-zealous therapist.

And Laura wasn't alone. Over the years, I've known countless students and parents who told me they (or their child) couldn't be on time or finish assignments because of their anxiety. Colleagues who reported they stole or couldn't tell the truth because they act uncontrollably under stress. I've snapped at my own kids or yelled at a car in traffic and blamed the anxiety.

None of this was true.

Sure, I had anxiety. And I was also a jerk.

Sure, people were desperately worried and chronically stressed. *But they chose* to lie or steal or cheat on their spouse.

Sure, you're always busy, always under pressure, and you have a lot of people reporting to you. But this isn't a license to shut the system down.

An anxiety diagnosis is not a new name. It's not a new identity. It doesn't describe who you are or even predict who you will be. An anxiety diagnosis simply means your body has been trying to get your attention in a particular way for a particular period of time. It's something you experience within the course of life as a normal, functioning human being. Yes, sometimes the experience is deeply painful, disruptive, or even devastating. Sometimes the alarms get out of whack and have to be recalibrated.

But you are not your anxiety.

With the right support, mentoring, and a good plan, you can teach your body that while you are indeed facing serious threats that need attention, you are safe and equipped to grow through whatever challenges come your way. You will learn to trust your body's alarm systems, possibly for the first time in your life.

If you've been diagnosed with some type of anxiety, obsessive-compulsive, or stress-related disorder, exhale. You now have some insight into how your body is trying to keep you safe. Insight and awareness are a great place to start on the path.

Medication Is Not the Only Answer for Anxiety

I'll begin with three truths:

1. I know this is a contentious, thin-ice topic.
2. Anxiety medication saved my life.
3. Anxiety medication did not heal or cure me.

Let's dig in.

I ignored my alarms for years. I said yes to everything, had zero boundaries, was in debt to the tune of hundreds of thousands of dollars, and never slept. I spent excessive energy ruminating on catastrophic thoughts, I gossiped, ran my mouth, and disconnected from my friend community. Eventually my alarms were ringing all the time. About everything. They were so loud I couldn't focus or hear anything else. Retreating into a shell of myself, I stuck my fingers in my ears.

I wasn't a failure or a loser. I wasn't broken, but my alarms had become far too sensitive.

My doctor ultimately recommended I take some anxiety medication, not so I would be healed or cured, but to help turn down the alarms *so I could do the work I needed to do to be well.* The work I needed to do included healing my marriage, making decisions about my career, finding community, taking a true inventory of my finances, and discerning the necessary steps to improve my environment.

I'll never forget the night I sat at my kitchen table with the pharmacy bag and its contents scattered in front of me. As I took that first pill, I wept and wept. I felt like a failure. A loser. A dad that my son could never be proud of. I felt so bad that my wife had chained herself to me.

My feelings, of course, weren't telling me the truth. The truth was, I had tried to manhandle my alarms on my own. I was unable to think, flex, or outwork my alarm systems. I needed to be honest about needing some support. By partnering with my doctor, I was taking courageous, brave steps into the heart of the storm.

Here are the facts about anxiety medications that I think are most helpful for our conversation:

1) *Anti-anxiety medications do not cure anxiety. They help manage symptoms.* People who are experiencing anxiety may be prescribed medications ranging from anti-depressants

to anti-seizure/anti-convulsants, anti-psychotics, antihistamines, and neuropeptides, to name a few broad categories. Each of these medicines are fraught with opportunities and challenges. They only work in a percentage of people, sometimes they have gnarly side effects (weight gain, sleepiness, decreased sexual function or desire, and so on), and the dosages generally have to be increased over time to keep up their anti-anxiety properties. As I've consumed more and more of the scientific literature and spoken with increasing numbers of mental-health and medical professionals, the general consensus is that when it comes to anxiety medications, prescribers can't guarantee how well they will work, which medications will help which patients, or for how long.

2) *Medications can be a powerful tool for creating a non-anxious life.* I cannot stress this enough. Medications did wonders for me and for many of the people I have walked alongside over the years. But they didn't suddenly make me not-anxious. They gradually turned down the alarms. They served as a flashlight in the dark—allowing me to see my way to the gym, to mindfulness, to health and healing, and to a counselor.

If you are currently taking anxiety medications, **DO NOT** immediately stop taking them. This is a dangerous and ill-advised decision. It's important to work with your doctor and wean off medications in an intentional fashion, when the time is right. Simply dropping certain medications can send shockwaves through your mind and body. Don't do this.

When it was time, I worked with my doctor to develop a step-wise plan to slowly decrease and discontinue my medications in conjunction with the other changes I was making in my life. This isn't a pass/fail assignment. It is a bumpy, start/stop transition. There's no race to some finish line. The goal here is a healthy, good life.

Some days it will feel impossible. You will think your body is failing you. You might also find that medications will be a part of your journey for a long, long time. In rare cases, you and your doctor may conclude that medication will be part of your life forever.

The main thing to remember is, the alarms are not the problem; the fire is the problem. If you continually avoid the alarms, or medicate them down so low that you can function without making changes, your house will burn down around you.

Medications can provide support as you choose to no longer hide from, avoid, or evade the fire.

For what it's worth, my personal rules for taking medication of any kind are threefold. First, I talk to one (or often more) medical professionals; I don't consult the internet. Second, I try all dietary, sleep, and physical interventions possible before I start trying pills. Third, I always have an end date in mind, a goal for getting off the medicine, before I put anything in my body.[28] I hold the end date loosely, knowing

---

[28] Of course, if I had a chronic illness or disease, I would gladly take medications for as long as necessary. If my doctor told me

that life happens. But it's important for me—and you—to go into interventions with intentionality and a plan. When I first began pharmacotherapy (the nerd word for taking medications), I committed to being on meds for up to six months. I ended up taking them longer, but it was important for me to have an initial check-in point before I took off down the road.

In all of it, I never forget I am in charge of my life and my body. Likewise, you are in charge of yours.

I work closely with my doctor and several other experts, but they know they are not in charge of my body. I am. I want to strongly encourage you to take ownership of your health in the same way.

This means that when I'm uncomfortable with something they are recommending, I tell them. I ask my doctors and counselors hard questions. When possible, I get multiple opinions.[29] I ask them what they are doing for themselves and for their kids. (This shows me what they *really believe*.) And I often request professional research and evidence for the interventions they're recommending—which they know I'll read! I'm not listening to the Instagram influencer *du*

---

my alarm system was permanently damaged, I'd happily take anti-anxiety medications until the end of time—grateful that I lived at a time in history when this is possible!

[29] Don't feel like you have to go to the ends of the earth for multiple opinions on every single issue, but if it's something important, seek out another expert opinion or two if you can.

jour. I'm not sourcing "secret information" from YouTube. I'm reading the studies directly, when possible.

At the same time, I'm not relying on my (often) limited understanding of the studies I'm reading. I rely on the expertise, observations, and personal experience of these professionals and what they're seeing in the other folks they're working with. As much as I refuse to pass the buck on my health, I also don't act like a reckless cowboy on things I don't fully understand. Ultimately, I am responsible for the choices I make about my body. But I am honest about what I don't know.

A final note on medications: The scientific literature regarding psychotropic medication—specifically anti-anxiety medications—is vast. There are countless journals, books, authors, and opinions. I respect the breadth of knowledge, and I have a ton to learn. I'm optimistic that advances in medicine will continue to improve our lives. But as I've said, anxiety medication is for support, not a cure. Medication can be an important and necessary part of the wellness journey. But in almost every case, it won't be the destination.

So if anxiety is not a disease, it's not a new identity, and if medication isn't the ultimate answer, then we find ourselves in need of new questions.

The questions are *not*: "What can I no longer do or enjoy now that I have anxiety?" or "How do I fix anxiety?" or "How do I cure anxiety?"

The new questions we need to ask are: "How do I build a non-anxious life where the alarms aren't ringing all the time?" and "How do I build a life that offers me peace, purposeful work, resilience, deep relationships, and joy?"

UNDECLARING CIVIL WAR ON OURSELVES

One thing we know about anxiety is that it narrows our field of focus. It makes us acutely aware of the perceived threats *coming at our own lives, right now.* Our vision constricts, our ability to think rationally or big-picture dissolves, and we become obsessed with survival. We're zoomed in on our belly button while the ceiling above us is caving in.

Everything in us gets tense. Scared. Life becomes us versus them—whoever *them* happens to be. And when we isolate ourselves long enough, the only enemy left is us. **We declare civil war. Against ourselves.** All our attention gets pointed inward. Almost without warning, it's you versus you.

And you're out for blood.

We go to war against our bodies and our thoughts and our feelings. We become obsessed with *my.* My life. My happiness. My truth. My pain. My annoyances. We begin to expect the world to cater to how we feel.

Let me be clear. Just like you, millions of people need the freedom to talk about their experiences and their pain. We all must learn to express our needs and reflect on our past traumas and present realities. There *is* injustice, evil, and abuse in this world that must be exposed and accounted for. But we also must be wary of letting these horrible moments or tragic experiences determine who we think we are. As if what happened to us in our darkest moments is all we will ever be.

This is deeply counter-cultural.

You and I have been told that our life is for one thing: self-actualization. That our destiny is in service of the perfected version of ourselves. We are obsessed with self-improvement. Self-governance. Self-reliance. Self, self, self. Or as Florida State professor, researcher, and suicideologist Thomas Joiner suggests, "soft-headed self-indulgence."

Discipline is critical. Hard work is a must. And personal growth is very important.

But personal growth makes a terrible god.

In our obsession with ourselves, our body sounds the alarms.

Anxiety narrows our focus. And the best place to hide, where no one can ever find us, is way inside ourselves.

Along the way, we try to capture and control anything we can. We video, photograph, and collect every concert, sunset, and memory of our kids inside four-inch metal boxes. We overschedule and overachieve and never stop moving, afraid we might miss out. And we regulate our lives with 72-degree homes and 72-degree cars and 72-degree offices as we hurriedly shuffle between each of them, never to go outside again. We become people we hate and we chain ourselves to anxious, anxious lives.

But there's another way.

Peace.

WHAT IS PEACE, ANYWAY?

My wife and I recently attended the funeral of one of my favorite cousins. He was older than me, but we looked just the same. We shared mannerisms, an off-color sense of humor, and an uncanny knack for getting ourselves in and out of trouble. Every time I saw him, he pulled me aside privately and told me he was proud of me.

And he passed away, sleeping next to his new wife, on a cruise ship.

No one was prepared for that phone call.

Or any call for that matter.

None of us are ever ready for the hard, gritty realities of life. The divorce. The abuse. Dad leaving. Your company closing.

But those calls will keep coming.

One day, about 10 years ago, I stopped doing what I'd always done.

I stopped running, stopped fighting, stopped pretending, and I turned and headed directly toward the Wizard behind the curtain.

I opened my hands.

I got humbled.

I paid off my debts.

Slowly but surely.

I healed some relationships, moved on from a few painful ones, and worked to begin adding new ones.

I started taking care of my mind, my body, my marriage, and my soul.

Lots of setbacks, but overall I kept moving forward.

And when my cousin died, I wasn't anxious. I had money in an emergency fund for a moment just like this. I bought plane tickets for me and my wife, and I never worried. We got a hotel room so we didn't have to sleep on some fourth cousin's living room floor on a makeshift pallet.

I'd been walking into the storm for years for just this moment.

And because I wasn't anxious—about the funeral, the family gathering, the finances, or my relationship with my cousin—I was able to feel the truest feeling in my body.

I was just sad.

Really, really sad.

I wept. I swore. I spent a long time talking to my cousin while he laid there in his casket. And my body stayed with me. It didn't run off into the woods, hiding from the grief or looking for future problems for future John to start solving. I didn't start fights with the family. I was able to just be really sad.

Exactly as I should have been.

Now make no mistake. For every moment like this that I get right, I'm working through countless other not-so-peaceful situations. But this painful time let me know I'm on the right path.

A peaceful life isn't drama-free or pain-free. A peaceful life refers to how you're able to handle things when they do indeed fall apart.

PEACE IS . . .

After decades of continuous war, several economic crises, a media industry obsessed with inciting panic, social media chaos, and political mayhem, we don't even know what peace looks or feels like.

In our frenetic, chaotic lives, peace sounds like something nostalgic, like your grandma's black-and-white photos or your stepdad's record collection. Or we think of it as just some buzzword stitched into pillows and murmured by hippies on organic llama farms. I want to reimagine peace and paint a crystal-clear picture for us to hold on to as we navigate the rough waters ahead.

Peace isn't something that just happens. Peace is a paradox in that we have to both go get it and accept it. We must take courageous, decisive action and we must open our hands and receive it. Peace is both disciplined hard work and a gift.

Peace is a choice.

Whether you knew it or not, that's why you picked up this book.

You want peace.

Peace is a good, deep night's sleep.

Peace is feeling appropriately stressed, but not anxious, about your job, your kids, or your spouse.

Peace is having close relationships that allow you to dream, ask hard questions, laugh from your gut, and feel both safe and passionate.

Peace is financial security.

Peace is being ambitious and driven yet understanding that no one can accumulate or accomplish their way to love or connection or joy.

Peace is going all-in on that next degree or first-place trophy—and knowing that when you achieve it, your dad still might not call and tell you he's proud of you.

Peace is telling the truth. Always. And being fully known and loved anyway.

Peace is not yelling at your kids or berating your spouse.

Peace is moving out of your home because he won't stop hitting you . . . and you have a safe place to go and financial resources to get you started on next steps.

Peace is walking out the door of a toxic workplace because you refuse to spend another minute in a gossipy, abusive environment. Or peace is staying put and enduring hardship because you have a greater mission, like transformative organizational change and safety for other employees.

Peace is trust.

Peace is a choice.

A NON-ANXIOUS LIFE

So here we are.

We know what anxiety is, what it isn't, and what it looks like in the wild.

And now it's time to get to work.

We've got miles to go before we sleep.

Here's where we're headed:

Building a non-anxious life is about becoming anti-fragile[30]—creating a life that actually grows and thrives during times of great distress and upheaval.

Building a non-anxious life is about being honest about what's coming. Something is always heading our way. Car accidents. Weather disasters. Illness. Family divisions.

There will always be fires and storms and dragons, especially the ones you don't see coming.

Building a non-anxious life is about being focused on controlling what I can control—and nothing more. And all I can control are *my* thoughts and *my* actions.

Someday the fires and storms and dragons will reach my front door. To help counter them, I can vote, get solar panels, build a tornado shelter, and teach my children what to do during an active-shooter event. Still, I can't be everywhere all the time or counteract every bad thing that will happen. And I rest here, knowing I'm doing what I can—and holding everything else loosely.

This is the non-anxious life.

And that's why you're here with me: you want to be free.

As we think through the choices we have to make to experience a non-anxious life, know this:

I don't care if you're a police officer,

---

[30] Nassim Nicholas Taleb's *Antifragile: Things That Gain from Disorder* (New York: Random House, 2014) is one of the most important books I've ever read. The rare masterpiece and paradigm shifter.

a lawyer,

a servicewoman returning from your third deployment,

a divorcee with two kids,

someone struggling in deep poverty or with heavy addiction,

a physician,

a minister,

or a hard-working dad just trying to untangle the world you've been told you must have from the world you actually want.

You are worth a non-anxious life.

You can choose it, create it, sustain it, and share it.

In order to build this kind of life, you will have to learn some new skills and consider some difficult changes. For some of you, these changes will be minor and simple. For many of us, including me, it will cost us our entire way of life.

I've seen countless men and women before you do it. I've been there too.

When you're ready, let's go.

THE
6 DAILY CHOICES

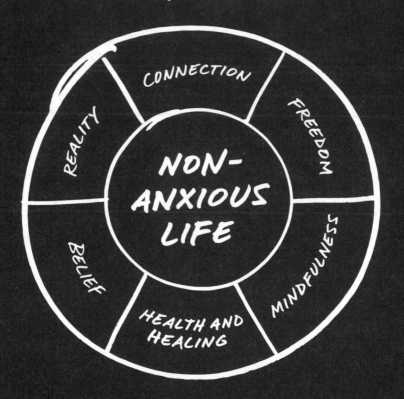

THE SIX DAILY CHOICES OF THE NON-ANXIOUS LIFE

So you're ready to build a non-anxious life?

It's going to be difficult. If you're not up for it, it's not too late to turn back.

It's going to require you to stop running. To turn where you are standing and face what's been chasing you. To head toward the fire.

Fires like the childhood abuse.

When your professor said you'd never make it.

How the government tells you how broken, maligned, and weak you are.

How your mom said you were ugly, unlovable, and unworthy.

The losses. The heartbreaks. The lost jobs. The piles of stuff everywhere you turn.

The things you saw at war. The addictions. The perfectionism. The loneliness. Your poor health or massive debt load. Your changing beliefs.

All of it.

You're going to have to turn and face it. And when you're ready, we'll walk right through the middle of it . . . together.

Think of the Six Daily Choices as a way of experiencing and interacting with the world.

You'll be good at a few of them, and they will come naturally to you. They'll be your go-to. Other choices will be tough, but not impossible. They will push you, but they won't be hard to implement. You'll take them on easily enough. Several choices will be agonizing to regularly incorporate into your life. Brutal, even. These choices will make you feel uncomfortable, scared, and incompetent. You'll have to learn new and different ways of doing life.

As you dig into each chapter, keep note of sections that make you think, *Impossible!* or *This is stupid!* or *There's no way I can do this!*

This may be where your dragons lie in wait.

OVER AND OVER AGAIN

The Six Daily Choices are not one-and-done. They're decisions you'll make—some minute by minute, some decade by decade—that will put you in a position to be resilient in the face of adversity. To roll with, or even take, the punches when they come. To get back up when you get knocked down. And believe me, you will get knocked down. It's just a matter of when.

Many people want to think they can avoid making choices.

They're convinced they can run from responsibility, or the work involved in building a non-anxious life.

Let me make this clear: You are making choices every day. And these choices are either creating an anxious world or a non-anxious one.

You get to choose.

You think you can avoid discomfort by not choosing. But as the mighty band Rush sang, this is also a choice.

THE BIG SIX

The Six Daily Choices are:

1. Choose Reality
2. Choose Connection
3. Choose Freedom
4. Choose Mindfulness
5. Choose Health and Healing
6. Choose Belief

These choices are not linear. I've illustrated them with a wheel because they don't start or stop in any order. They work in sync with each other. Of course, there will be days, or even seasons, when one or more of these choices is incredibly challenging or intentionally gets put on the backburner. That's okay. We're trying to build a different kind of life, not win some sort of existential contest.

As I said above, some of you will find an easy entrance into the Six Daily Choices by paying off your debts and cleaning out the clutter from your lives. Others will find entry through their counselor or care group, their workout program, or separating from a toxic relationship. Others will get sick of being alone and reach out to an old friend.

Some of you will always take the stairs. Never owe anyone money. Learn to control your thoughts and create space between stimulus and response. Others will rest deeply in their anchor to a higher power. The belief in something bigger than themselves.

You can enter wherever you want. But you can't cut corners or skip over steps. This isn't Candyland.

And because it's represented as a wheel, think of it this way: being out of balance in one area will eventually pull your entire life out of alignment. You'll know you're out of alignment when you find yourself anxious, burned out, or stressed beyond comprehension.

You can have great relationships and a great therapist, yet be in an abusive, unsafe work environment . . . and your body will sound the alarms.

You can have a great job and strong friendships, and yet have a dysregulated relationship with food, too much debt, and be buried in endless amounts of junk in your home and digital life . . . and your body will sound the alarms.

You can have the best abs in the world, more money than anyone you know, and try to maintain your position as the center of the world . . . and your anxiety alarms will ring off the wall.

You've been making choices all along and you didn't even realize it.

It's time to try something completely new.

ALONE, TOGETHER

If you decide to move on to chapter 4, it's game on.

Writing this book changed me, and I knew what was coming. Most of you will never be able to see the world the same way again. This is what I'm aiming for.

For some of you, the Six Daily Choices will cause you to rethink, reexamine, and ultimately change much about your life. Some of you will reimagine everything. For others, you'll realize you're out of whack in a few areas, but doing well everyplace else.

Everyone will have areas where they can dig in and find more peace. Some by working harder, others by letting go. I'll walk you through each step along the way.

Before we go, internalize these two truths:

No one can make you head into the storm.

No one.

Not your spouse, your kids, your boss. Not your friends, your mentor, or your pastor.

You must make this decision on your own.

Also, you can't head into the storm alone. It's too strong. It's wiped out many before you who were smarter, stronger, and better equipped.

Where two or more are gathered, the anchor holds.
You're tethered in, ready to head out.
If you're ready to build a non-anxious life, turn the page.
This is where everything changes.

THE
6 DAILY CHOICES

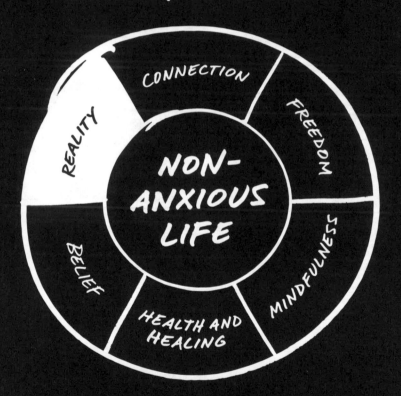

CHAPTER 4

CHOOSE REALITY

I once met with a woman who was worried about her marriage. I'll call her Dana.

Dana and her husband had been married for about a decade. She told me she'd had an ongoing affair with a work colleague for almost a year before eventually being caught by her husband. Her husband was understandably heartbroken, they legally separated, and he moved out of their home.

After some months of separation, both Dana and her husband decided to try and rekindle their relationship. They went to counseling, started dating a bit, and were making a run at healing their marriage.

Dana was constantly haunted by the fact that she'd done something she had never thought herself capable of: cheating on her husband. She was all-in on trying to save her marriage. Each little step toward reconciliation helped her breathe a little easier. She wanted her marriage to work.

The rekindling continued for months and then, some-what abruptly, her husband stopped returning calls. He quit responding to text messages. He didn't move back in. One of his buddies told Dana that he'd seen him on a few dates with another woman. When Dana would show up at his apart-ment to pick up or drop off their daughter, they would talk briefly, but there was no warmth or connection—only the perfunctory exchanging of information.

Dana was grasping at a ghost.

She told me she wasn't sleeping at night. She was anx-ious, frustrated, and feeling out-of-control. Like falling but unable to see the ground. She had sought me out to figure out how to encourage her husband to keep working on their marriage. What could she do to get him to start returning calls? What could she say to reignite his passion? Dana was desperately looking for some missing puzzle piece.

There was a heavy pause between us while I waited for her to feel the weight of her words. Words she had thought but never spoken aloud before.

The silence felt like a fog.

As compassionately as I could, I quietly said, "Dana . . . your marriage is over."

Tears streamed down her face.

After a brief moment, I asked, "Am I right?"

"Yes," she said through tears.

I continued, "Behavior is a language. Your husband, in his own cowardly, avoidant way, is telling you everything you need to know. He has decided he is done being married to you, and now it's a question of who has the courage to take this thing off life support."

Dana cried. Hard.

I got choked up too.

Now to be clear, this was a short meeting between strangers. I've seen marriages on the brink like hers be restored. For her and her husband to heal their marriage wasn't impossible—but it was very unlikely. It would take a radical recommitment from both. It would take long-term, continued, unified work, almost certainly with professional therapists. And in our short conversation, I didn't hear anything of the sort. I heard the opposite.

The next move was going to be Dana's. She had to choose to stare down reality so that her brain, body, and spirit could begin to sift through the chaos and figure out the most terrifying question that most of us spend our lives avoiding:

"What am I going to do now?"

WE'RE ALWAYS SOLVING FOR REALITY

When I was a kid, one of my favorite movies was *Bill and Ted's Excellent Adventure*. I must have watched it a thousand times. It's about two knuckleheaded friends who are failures at both school and their dream of becoming rockstars. They're quietly watching their lives flush down the drain when someone from the future (Rufus, played brilliantly by George Carlin) shows up to help them pass high school so they can be about their true mission: saving the planet and ushering in world peace, all through the power of their rock 'n' roll.[31]

Bill and Ted end up time-traveling in an old phone booth, gathering people of historical significance for a final school project. They manage to kidnap Abraham Lincoln, Genghis Kahn, Sigmund Freud, Beethoven, and Joan of Arc, among others. As they fly about through time and space, multiple versions of Bill and Ted are spun off into different strands of time, kind of like *Back to the Future* meets *Tommy Boy* meets *Being John Malkovich*.

At one critical juncture in the film, Rufus tells Ted, "Don't forget to wind your watch." Rufus goes on to explain to Bill and Ted that as they are traveling through time, having adventures and meeting people, the clock in their hometown is still ticking away. They might be having experiences and escapades in far-off lands, but they are still anchored to reality at home.

The clock in San Dimas, Rufus says, is always ticking.

I was reminded of this story when I was first introduced to Dr. Bessel van der Kolk's book *The Body Keeps the Score*.[32]

---

[31] The movie was ridiculous, and I don't even care. Be excellent to each other.

[32] I know, I know, there probably aren't a lot of folks who read *The Body Keeps the Score* (New York: Penguin Books, 2014) and immediately thought of *Bill and Ted's Excellent Adventure*, but alas . . . this is why I live in the woods and don't have a lot of friends.

The ticking clock in San Dimas reminded me of our individual minds, bodies, and spirits. Because no matter where we go, how successful we are, how much money we make, how beautiful our spouse is, how many walls we build in and around our lives to protect us, or how many books we read, *our body is always keeping score.* Our brain is always scanning the world around us for threats and dangers, often informed by past experiences, with the goal of keeping us alive. Our body is always sounding the alarms.

Your body knows how well you are, regardless of how you try to numb it or lie to it.

As I've studied and written on acute and secondary trauma, discovered more about how our nervous system works, met with expert researchers and practitioners, and walked with people through brutal, grief-filled moments, I've come to believe one critically important thing: **Our bodies are constantly solving for reality, even if we are not**.

Makeup can hide scars, but the scars remain. Bandages can cover up wounds, but the wounds still exist. We can wear masks, feel pity, create distance, or pretend things are different than they are, but our body is keeping the score.

Your body knows if you're in an unsafe and abusive relationship, even if he keeps telling you he loves you.

Your body knows you're broke and dangerously close to a financial cliff, even as you emotionally numb yourself buying garbage you don't need to impress people you don't like.

Your body knows your small business is failing, even if you haven't looked at your profit-and-loss statements for months.

Your body knows your wife is quickly flipping the phone face-down every time you walk into the room, even if you're lying to yourself that she's just chatting with her girlfriends.

And when your brain and body believe you're not safe, it will sound the alarms.

CHOICE ONE

The first choice toward building a non-anxious life is honesty. Honesty with yourself and with others.

You must *Choose Reality.*

Choosing reality is the practice of taking a true inventory of your life, your work, your relationships, and your values. Best-selling author, professor, and educational advocate Dr. Parker Palmer describes it as stepping back from viewing our lives in tiny slivers to see the "profound truth."[33] Former Navy Seal and best-selling author Jocko Willink calls it "ownership."[34] My friend's dad called it "starin' down the devil."

This is facing the truth.

You have to choose to live in truth, however painful and ugly it might be. Choosing reality is where all healing and change begins.

---

[33] Parker J. Palmer, *The Courage to Teach: Exploring the Inner Land-scape of a Teacher's Life* (San Francisco: Wiley, 2017), 65.
[34] Jocko Willink, *Discipline Equals Freedom: Field Manual* (New York: St. Martin's Press, 2020), 19.

THE TWO SIDES

When it comes to creating a non-anxious life, there are two sides of facing reality: the dark side and the light side. Let's explore them both below.

The dark side is the scary or challenging reality that's staring you down. You've been hurt, your dreams are in ashes, and you must face the facts.

- Your dog is riddled with cancer and lost in pain.
- Your division at work is still losing money and layoffs are coming soon.
- Travel sports are consuming your weekends, your holidays, your money, and your lives.
- You bought way more house than you could afford and you're drowning in debt.
- Your husband said he wasn't talking to her anymore . . . but he keeps hiding his phone.
- Your mom is no longer healthy enough to live alone.
- You don't exercise, you don't sleep well, and your diet is 84 percent drive-thru.

This dark side of reality is about owning up to the ways your life has been impacted by trauma, and the ways it has changed, or is changing, negatively. The abuse. The debt. The pain. The abandonment. The 30 extra pounds. The world that's passing you by.

In addition to facing the dark things in life, we must also be honest about the good things. The light.

Many folks I walk alongside speak only of the darkness. They refuse to acknowledge the good and the beautiful things. They walk through life with their head down, refusing to see beauty and laughter and blessings. They ignore the ways the world is open to them.

But make no mistake: light and beauty can be found everywhere.

- Your spouse is your biggest fan, especially since you got laid off.
- Both of your children are healthy, silly, and full of energy.
- There is food in your fridge and you've never known true, paralyzing hunger.
- Your heater works in the winter.
- Sure, it's not your dream job and the leader is a goofball, but you have a good job, with a decent salary and health insurance for you and your family.
- You experienced abuse in the past, but you've learned tremendous grit, resilience, and most importantly, you're safe now.

When we're not honest about the light, we internalize and identify with the awful things that have been done to us: "Everybody has it out for me," or "I'm a victim of . . ." By choosing reality, we opt to look at the full spectrum of truth. The dark and the light.

In one situation, we're not looking at the darkness because we're terrified of what we'll see. In the other situation, we're unable or unwilling to acknowledge the light because our bodies are so locked into scanning for threats and preparing for the end of the world, we can't stop and smell anything, much less the roses.

And all the while, our anxiety alarms are ringing.

You're Not Broken and You're Not Crazy

If you've experienced painful loss—the loss of a loved one or a career or your home country—or you've experienced racism, deep poverty, or have been otherwise shoved to the margins, facing reality can be terrifying. Because in your life, reality *has been traumatizing.* This sort of reality bottoms us out. It feels like the ending (which in some cases it is). Your body *should* be trying to get your attention! The anxiety alarms mean your body is working properly.

Or, if you've spent your career hustling and earning enough money to create a comfortable life for your family, you might have also recognized that your wealth and achievement couldn't make your kids want to spend time with you. Your alarms may have been ringing for some time, even though it appears you have it all together.

As much as we want to pretend we can avoid reality, our bodies know.

I've seen high-profile teaching and research professors retire and clean out their offices. Their books end up in a Free—Take One pile in the hallway; their vacant job is posted before the end of the month. Our bodies know.

While our brains chase and achieve and accomplish, our bodies are trapped in reality.

RATIONALLY IRRATIONAL

Facing reality is both a philosophical and practical challenge. First, as best-selling authors and internationally renowned psychologists Dr. Dan Ariely and Dr. Daniel Kahneman have separately found in their studies, people are not rational beings. We act in ways that don't make sense. We're wired and taught to avoid things, make emotional, incorrect judgments, and otherwise act illogically. We inherently slow down and stare at the car wreck. Obsessively scroll for the next tragic headline. Keep meditating on the image of our son right after he broke his arm.

Our brain wants us to never forget the horrors of the world around us (remember the GPS pins from chapter 2). It wants us to always be ready for the next calamity. This protective nature makes sense, but it implies a sense of control over the world that you and I don't really have.

You didn't cause the car wreck.

Or the economic implosion.

Or your dad's exit.

So, our brains are often chasing solutions to unsolvable problems. And when it can't solve them in the past, it casts them into some unknown future. In this way, we are wired to be rationally irrational and sensibly foolish. Our bodies are sprinting on a hamster wheel to nowhere.

Additionally, we're stronger than we know and able to endure much more than we think we can. Which is how we're often able to plow through reality, pretending it doesn't apply to us. We've all managed, at one time or another, to push the consequences off into the future. Our bodies have built-in mechanisms that allow us to function in the face of great tragedy, hardship, or loss—for a while. We have protective psychological and physical abilities that make it possible for us to maintain some sort of equilibrium, often in stark denial of reality for a while, but at great cost to our long-term health and well-being. We'll die from smoking, obesity, and alcoholism . . . later.

I once had a friend tell me she became convinced her husband was cheating on her. But instead of simply asking him (he wasn't cheating, by the way), she chose to ignore it because she couldn't deal with the thought of what lay on the other side of infidelity. She just kept plowing ahead, pretending everything was fine, reality and anxiety alarms be damned. Years later, when the reality of the secrets, disconnection, accusations, and mistrust came to light, I watched my friend's marriage nearly supernova.

And this is the way most of us live. Ignoring. Pretending. Procrastinating. Waiting for motivation or feelings. Blaming things on everyone else. Or spitting at ourselves in the mirror. We ignore the light or the dark or both.

We avoid reality.

We just assume we can eat whatever we want, or never exercise or sleep. We pretend only other people get sick, or that we can max out our credit for a business idea with no alternative plan, and somehow it's all going to be okay.

As best-selling author Ryan Holiday points out, "Far too many people don't have a backup plan because they refuse to consider that something might not go exactly as they wish."[35] We spend time worrying about the apocalypse, but we don't have an emergency fund or a couple of friends to call in the middle of the night. And because of the extraordinary technological and societal advancements made in the past 200 years, we often don't have to face reality for long stretches of time.

DISTRACTED FROM REALITY

Truthfully, as the most distracted people in history, choosing reality is incredibly hard.

Why invest time and energy in a back-up plan, go get my blood drawn, or have a brutally hard conversation with my wife when I can spend hours on the latest app (or doing just about anything else for that matter)? It's just too easy to check out and look the other way. Instead of dealing with reality, we can scroll, surf, shop, and binge our way to numb indifference.

I'm not being defeatist. Yes, there are times to be courageous against enormous odds. History is built on those who

---

[35] Ryan Holiday, *The Obstacle Is the Way: The Timeless Art of Turning Trials into Triumph* (New York: Portfolio/Penguin, 2014), 140.

threw caution to the wind and went after the impossible. The Elon Musks and Steve Jobs of the world ignored reality and made magic . . . The Astros won the World Series without cheating . . . I get the impossible happening.

But these are wild outliers. Black swans.[36] Way, way, way outside the bell curve.

If we have tons of debt, no personal savings or emergency fund, and are dumping our time and money into speculative hacks like digital currencies, we're not living in reality. If we don't have friends and we don't have the skills to have a hard, loving conversation, we're playing make-believe. If our business is falling apart and we just keep tightening our grip on our employees and getting more and more angry, we're firing arrows at the wrong target.

And our body is keeping the score.

THE METEORITE PLAN

When I was in the dark depths of my season of anxiety, I was hard to be around. One time during this season, I sat down with my great friend Todd, a finance wizard from Texas. I was peppering him with a million questions about currency, state and federal solvency, bond rate impacts on debt ratios, and what we were going to do when the dollar goes to zero.

---

[36] Nassim Nicholas Taleb's masterpiece, *The Black Swan: The Impact of the Highly Improbable* (New York: Random House, 2008).

At some point he stopped me and told me something that changed my life. "You know, John, I don't have a meteorite plan."

"I don't get what you're saying," I responded.

He repeated, "I don't have a meteorite plan." Then he continued, "If the US dollar becomes worthless and the stock market disappears, you're going to be fighting your neighbor for their water. Your neighbor might try and steal your pets for food. I don't have a plan for that. Is investing risky? Of course. Is doing nothing risky? Of course. I'm going to look at the information I have, and make the best decisions I can moving forward. And after that, if we get hit by a meteorite, I'll deal with it when it happens."

Bam! It hit me right between the eyes. I was refusing to see the light. I was obsessed with fantasy in the dark.

Ever since that conversation, I've quietly found that the smartest and most successful men and women I know do not have an apocalypse plan. Not because they have a death wish, but because they understand there is little to plan for when the end of times arrives. Your Go Bag won't get you very far.

Now don't get me wrong: I do have a few deep freezers and a giant garden. I keep an eye on the meteorites. My good friend John is a former Navy Seal, and I call him when it looks like things are going to set off. But I don't walk around with my head in the clouds, holding my breath for the end of time.

Being non-anxious isn't about trying to ignore every unsavory and ugly thing. Avoiding the alarms makes them louder and stronger. Being non-anxious also isn't about imagining and trying to solve for each and every catastrophic scenario in my present life either. This is a fool's errand. A waste of time. A way to avoid meeting my neighbors, loving my family, and taking care of myself. We have to take care of the long tails[37] in either direction and we have to face our present reality.

LOVE BITES, AND REALITY HURTS

Real life is hard. It's every single day and it never stops. And then someone you love passes away or you learn your kid's diagnosis, and it gets even harder. Building a non-anxious life is about realizing: *reality hurts*. No amount of screaming and being angry is going to change the election results. Or give you your job back. Or convince your ex to return.

Choosing reality is owning that your kids didn't make you raise your voice. They don't have that kind of power. You were unprepared, tired, stressed, and impatient—and you took it out on them.

Choosing reality is knowing that the barista with 41 pieces of flare on his vest did not make you act rudely. He was just doing his job, poorly, and you lost it. You were already in a bad mood when you placed your order. You chose to act like a child. You made a choice.

---

[37] Long tails are a picture of statistical risk. Read Taleb's *The Black Swan*, 223–225, for an eloquent explanation.

Choosing reality is about taking responsibility for the food you eat. Or taking on a second and third job for 18 months and missing your kid's school plays and basketball games so you can finally pay off your debts.

And we could go on and on.

Choosing reality is about taking an inventory of the *challenges* in your life, your relationships, your family, your place in the world—and being honest about where you are versus where you wanted to be.

Choosing reality is also about taking an inventory of the *good things* in your life and being honest about how you ignore the good stuff and instead spend time worshiping the negative, soulless, ugly stuff. How you watch YouTube videos about Bigfoot instead of playing trains with your son. Or you stay glued to political-opinion shows instead of kicking the soccer ball with your daughter.

For millions and millions of us, when we drop our guard, stop running in anxious little circles, and take true inventory of our lives, reality can be devastating, heartbreaking and downright scary.

But to heal from anxiety, we must no longer avoid it or run around it.

We have to go through it.

THE ROLE OF GRIEF AND HIDING FROM HARDSHIP

In *Own Your Past, Change Your Future,* I wrote extensively about the critical importance of grief in the life of a healing, whole person. Grief involves experiencing sadness—sometimes as a shallow stream and sometimes as a raging sea. It's grueling and unpleasant, different for every single person, and we often head into grief without any game plan. Frankly, most of us just try to skip it, hoping it will go away.

One aspect of the anxious lives we've created for ourselves stems from our obsession with avoiding discomfort. With not wanting to feel bad. Or wanting to avoid the ugly cry, the hard conversation, or the fact that you can't afford to live in your city anymore.

Over the past few decades, we've found ourselves in a small sliver of history where basic needs such as food and shelter have been made widely available. This era of abundance has allowed us to disconnect ourselves from emotional realities like grief. Death. Frustration. Disappointment. We now have energy and space and distractions to escape being sad. And it's costing us our very souls.

As living standards have increased, we've moved our collective concerns away from trying to survive, to trying to be comfortable. At the same time, we have continued to increasingly pathologize discomfort. We've made what's uncomfortable or hard the enemy. And our alarms are sounding.

The Face of Grief

To create a non-anxious life, we must choose reality, and sometimes that means inviting sadness and grief as fellow travelers.

Reality, for all of us, will involve hurt.

Dr. George A. Bonanno, author and professor of psychology at Columbia University, notes what research groups have revealed: "with sadness comes accuracy."[38] Grief serves as a clarifying agent for the body. Bonanno adds, "Studies have shown that people made to feel sad are . . . more accurate in the way they view their own abilities and performance and are also more thoughtful and less biased in their perceptions of other people. . . . In general then, sadness helps us focus accurately and promotes deeper and more effective reflection."[39]

There is no non-anxious life without sadness. Without pain. Without discomfort. I have to choose to grieve these things alongside the heartbreaking, sometimes angering realities others face that make me feel weak. Powerless. Sad.

- Someone will break my son's heart. Someone will say something demoralizing and ugly to my daughter. Someone will steal from my family, lie about me on the internet, or make a decision that hurts people I love.
- Someone I'm close to will be diagnosed with terminal cancer, or dementia, or some other disease, and nothing I do will be able to save them.

---

[38] George A. Bonanno, *The Other Side of Sadness: What the New Science of Bereavement Tells Us About Life After Loss* (New York: Basic Books, 2019), 45.
[39] Bonanno, *The Other Side of Sadness*, 46–47.

- Someone I despise will get elected president. There will be famines and wars and rumors of war, earthquakes and oil spills and floods.

This is the truth. This is reality.

But here's what is amazing.

On the other side of grief is *action*: the discovery of meaning, or sometimes the creation of it. It's deciding where we go from here. It's gathering a tribe around you, making a plan, and taking one tiny, wobbly step in a new direction.

On the other side of grief is *exhale*. There is a great relief in accepting reality.

On the other side of grief is *compassion*. We find grace. And that grace extends to ourselves and to those around us.

On the other side of grief is *boldness*. I can look into the darkness, surrounded by people I love and trust, and head toward the light. I can believe. I can hope. I can search for beauty once again.

I can choose reality.

Living in the Paradox: Controlling What We Can Control

As we close out this chapter, I want to make one thing crystal clear: We don't make good decisions when we're scared. Or alone. Or anxious. Or depressed. Or drunk. In fact, when we're in fight, flight, or freeze, our brain doesn't want us to waste precious resources on rational thought.

It just wants us to RUN! Or DEFEND! Or PLAY DEAD!

Best-selling author and Franciscan mystic Richard Rohr explains, "Yes, the mind and reason are necessary, but they must learn to distinguish between what lies beyond its reach. Yes, the mind is brilliant, but the more we observe it, the more we see it is also obsessive and repetitive."[40]

Now that we understand this, let me offer two critically important steps for choosing reality.

First, as we're setting about to change our life, we can't do it by ourselves. I'm a born-and-bred Texas male. Trust me, I've tried. Staring at your own soul, all by yourself, is like staring at the sun. It's beautiful and scary, and it will make you blind.

I've found that the only way I'm able to choose and see reality in most instances is to have someone with me. A friend, a mentor, a counselor, a minister, a coach. I need other people.

The other step toward choosing reality is a baseline inventory. When my good friend Dr. Layne Norton was helping me with some nutritional goals, he told me: "If you don't measure it, you can't change it." Turns out, the reality of how many calories I was eating was different from how many I thought I was eating. In the immortal words of Lloyd Christmas, "I was way off . . ."

---

[40] Richard Rohr, *The Naked Now: Learning to See as the Mystics See* (New York: Crossroad, 2009), 55.

When taking a reality inventory, we have to look at the details *and* we have to step back and measure the landscape, looking for patterns, shadows, and patches of light. You want to recognize: How good is my marriage, really? How much weight have I gained? How severed is my relationship with my daughter? How little do I actually sleep? You have to stare both into the light and into the void.

So let's buckle in, get out both our magnifying glass and our telescope, and gather our people around us. Let's choose reality.

CHOOSE REALITY

Chapter Summary and Next Steps

Summary:

- You must choose to face reality. Reality is your starting line for charting a new course.
- Choosing reality is the only way your brain, body, and spirit can begin to sift through what is true, what is false, and what you are going to do about it.
- Taking an inventory of the *challenges* in your life, your relationships, your family, your health, your station in life—and being honest about where you are versus where you wanted to be—will help you identify the gap between what you desire your life to look like and the reality of where it is now.

- In addition to facing the dark things in life, we must also be honest about the good things. The light. The beauty and laughter and blessings.
- To heal from anxiety, we must no longer avoid it or run around it. We have to go through it.

Things to Do:

- Create space to take inventory of your life, your work, your relationships, and your values. *Set aside time for this journaling exercise.* Put time on the calendar and hold to it.
- **Download the *Choose Reality journaling template* at johndelony.com/resources** or pull out an old notebook. It's time to write down FACTS about these key areas of your life. Be honest.

Relationships

- What is the state of my marriage?
- What is my relationship with my kids?
- What is my relationship with my co-workers?
- How is my relationship with my parents? Siblings?
- How many close friends do I have?

Health

- Am I overweight? How many medications am I taking?
- Do I have chronic pain, illness, and/or stress?
- How do I eat? Do I honor my body?
- How often do I consume alcohol?

- Do I exercise and incorporate challenging physical movement into my daily life?

Money

- How much debt do I owe?
- How much cash do I have in the bank?
- How much do I have saved for retirement?
- What is my relationship with money?
- Do I have—or am I on track to have—enough money to retire?

Career

- Do I have purpose in my work?
- Do I look forward to starting work each day?
- Is my work challenging and appropriately difficult to keep me inspired and engaged?
- Am I compensated fairly for what I do?
- Is my work environment contributing to or detracting from my overall emotional and physical health?
- Does my work matter?

Ask Yourself:

- What are some areas of my life that are going well?
- What are some areas of my life I would like to change?
- Do I like myself? Am I proud of the person I am and who I am becoming?
- Do I like how I feel? Do I like how I look?
- Am I a good spouse/friend/community member?

Additional Resources:

- Go to johndelony.com/resources for a list of books, podcasts, and tools to help you start down the path toward a non-anxious life.

THE
6 DAILY CHOICES

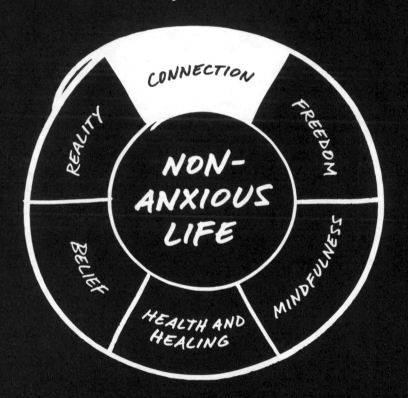

CHAPTER 5

CHOOSE CONNECTION

If the sky that we look upon
Should tumble and fall
Or the mountains should crumble to the sea
I won't cry, I won't cry
No, I won't shed a tear
Just as long as you stand
Stand by me.

Ben E. King, Jerry Leiber, and Mike Stoller,
"Stand By Me" (1962)

When I first began hosting a listener-call-in show and podcast, I was stunned that people would actually call a stranger and open up about their sex lives, addictions, special-needs children, family tragedies, and mental-health diagnoses.

In the beginning, I often blurted out without thinking, "Why in the world are you calling me with such a personal question? I'm just a clown on a podcast—you don't even know me!"

And practically every time, the response was the same: "Man, I've got no one else to call."

I've had those moments too. Like the day I learned that *Own Your Past, Change Your Future* hit number-one on the bestseller list. I found out when I was headed to a book signing; it was surreal and pretty cool. A small gang of us were in the car—the core team who had worked tirelessly to get my new book out into the world. We cheered, stopped for some champagne, and headed over to the bookstore.

A few people from work called to congratulate me. Those were wonderful calls.

I called my wife and mom and let them know.

And then I called . . .

No one.

I don't know why. My closest friends would have been thrilled to hear the news. But I just chickened out.

I did the book signing and hung out with people until late. Back at the hotel, I put on some shorts and a t-shirt and sat quietly by myself. I have great, wonderful friends. The best of the best. I've known some of these people for a few decades or more. But over the previous weeks, I had holed myself up behind my computer screen—writing, editing, putting out blogs and articles, and doing countless media hits. I was super-busy with work, my show, with book edits, as well as my kids and my wife. And the holidays were chaotic, and then I was on the road.

What had started out as several weeks of a packed schedule turned into six months. For some of my friends, six months had turned into more than a year. And it felt ridiculous to pick up the phone and begin calling folks I hadn't talked to in all that time and declare, "This great thing just happened for me!"

And so I sat on my hotel bed for a bit longer. I set my phone down, brushed my teeth, and tried to sleep.

I hoped someone would call. Not surprisingly, no one did.

RUNNING TO FILL THE VOID

For millions of us, this is our life. We get busy, we get married, we move. Then the first divorce happens in your friend group, the first kid, and we transition from hanging out every day to once a month to long running text threads. From by-my-side best friend to person-I-send-memes-to.

We keep meaning to reach out. To call and check in.

But we don't.

And almost overnight, as a culture, we've become so, so lonely. With little warning, we're asking ourselves to do something we have never, ever done before. We're asking our bodies, minds, and spirits to manage everything, all alone.

We're on our own.

And no, this isn't woo-woo garbage or political propaganda or over-spiritualization. This is neuroscience and cognitive psychology and common sense.

To build a non-anxious life, you have to choose to invite other people into your life. Knee to knee and shoulder to shoulder. You have to choose openness. You have to choose awkwardness. You have to choose to not live a life of isolation.

You must *Choose Connection*.

SURVEY SAYS . . .

In 2022, the research team at Ramsey Solutions did a massive study into the mental health, relationships, and well-being of thousands and thousands of Americans.[41] Here are some of the things we found:

82 percent of people say that those they spend the most time with don't know them deeply. Wow. Eight out of 10 of you are hanging out with people who don't know that you're struggling with your faith, or with your weight, or that you aren't attracted to your spouse anymore. Or that you are desperately worried about your daughter getting bullied or whether you'll be able to keep the house.

68 percent say they have three or fewer close friends. Don't miss this. Almost 7 out of 10 of you say you have three or fewer close friends. These are folks you'd call if your dad was having surgery. Or your car broke down. Or if you were out

---

[41] "The State of Mental Health," Ramsey Solutions (2022).

of town and your phone notified you that the water main in your home has burst. This is who you call when you need somewhere to turn.

More than half (54 percent) of the respondents reported they don't have a friend they feel comfortable calling in the middle of the night for an emergency. This one is a punch in the gut.

Half of you have no one to call, even in case of an emergency. Imagine your body laying down to sleep every night and the deep-seated part of your brain responsible for keeping you alive looks around and recognizes you have nobody to help you out if you're overcome with a full-blown asthma attack. Or if you were to slip coming out of the bathroom at 4:00 a.m. It's like waking up to find yourself with no place to call home. Or no insurance. Or no emergency fund. This is you without a safety net, and your body knows it.

Like it or not: **Other people are your emergency fund for life.**

Hardships and emergencies *will* come knocking at your door. And when you have no one to call, your brain will never let you rest. It will constantly be sounding the alarms.

Nearly half (47 percent) of married couples admit to struggling with sexual intimacy, and 40 percent struggle with emotional intimacy with their spouse. This data point lodged itself deep in my soul.

With our spouse, we have made long-term plans together. We share a home, a bed, and a life. In many cases, we've raised (or are raising) kids together. We sit with each other through our parent's cancer, through job loss, and through illnesses. We co-parent, co-earn, and co-manage everything. Yet despite this, we don't know how to say:

"I need more from our sex life."

"I don't like it when you do that."

"I need additional help from you around the house and with the kids."

"You are more connected to your phone than to me, and I'm beginning to look for affirmation in other people."

This goes far beyond having difficult conversations. This is about our souls turning to dust as we shop for new cars, build retirement plans, and review college applications.

Almost overnight in our world, we can't talk to people we love, much less our neighbors or strangers. We have few or no close friends. We have almost no middle-of-the-night friends. We can't even tell our spouses what we need. We are around people all day, but we're alone in a crowded room.

You know why 40-year-old guys get together for cookouts and cigars and still recount their football stories from high school? Or that one concert we all went to, that time Mike missed out on hooking up with so-and-so, or the deer that Justin almost got with his bow? You know why the BFFs still plan an overnight getaway and laugh their heads off about Brittany's wild bachelorette party, or that ski trip you all took over spring break in 2004? You ever wonder why your friends and colleagues who are military veterans or former first responders always get together and share war stories or near-misses?

Because that was the last time they were a part of something bigger than themselves.

It was the last time any of us belonged.

After that, we set off to do life alone.

THE PRISONER'S PUNISHMENT

When a prisoner violates the rules of their jail, they are sent to isolation. The hole. After a judge and jury have removed a person's freedoms and locked him or her away, there is still one more punishment that can be dished out.

They pull him or her from the presence of other prisoners and make them spend time alone. Completely alone.

Some psychological researchers consider isolation a form of torture.

And now this is all of us. We're doing this to ourselves.

Have you ever sat at a table of family and friends, surrounded by people who care about you—maybe at a reunion, a big work event, a baby shower, or a church potluck—and felt like you were absolutely alone? Have you ever grabbed your phone for the hundredth time and realized still no one has texted you? Or you have 29 text messages all asking you for something . . . but nobody is checking in on you? Ever fold your laptop for the day after working from home and realize you didn't hear the voice of anyone who wasn't on a podcast?

This is the world we've created.

THE LONELINESS ALARMS

How does being lonely connect to anxiety?

As we've discussed, our brains are constantly scanning our environments for threats. Whether or not we are consciously paying attention, our brains are monitoring for people, things, or situations that can take us out. And when we're lonely, the body ramps up threat detection. It raises the baseline threat level because it knows one critical fact: *You're out here by yourself.* You can't rely on your tribe to spot danger, and you have no one else to build a fire or to gather food while you're keeping watch.

You're on your own—and your body knows it.

When your brain identifies that you're all alone, it dumps cortisol and adrenaline into the bloodstream: *This is a problem you must solve NOW!*

This is an emergency! A crisis! Sound the alarms!

There is activation across our HPA (hypothalamic-pituitary-adrenal) axis. Glucocorticoids are released into the bloodstream, affecting multiple organ systems, in order to prepare the body for war.

Here's something else: When our brain recognizes we're alone, it divides up the world into *us* and *them.* Who's safe and who's not. It overidentifies people and situations as threatening because, when solving for survival, it's better to assume something is a threat and be wrong—and still be alive—than to ignore something and get killed.

Being lonely makes us feel and see threats that aren't

really there. Threats that don't exist in reality. Nevertheless, feelings and emotions begin to overwhelm our body, in addition to the other ways our body tries to get our attention. Suddenly, we're a ball of anxiety and panic.

Researchers such as John Cacioppo, Louise Hawkley, Sarah Pressman, and countless others have painted a clear yet terrifying picture of loneliness.

Loneliness increases your risk of:

- heart attacks
- cardiovascular disease
- cancer
- addiction
- Alzheimer's and dementia
- depression
- personality disorders
- suicidal ideation
- yelling at the high school kid who is umpiring your son's Little League game

And no, I don't care if you've taken some online quiz that claimed you're an introvert. I don't care what your Enneagram number is. And yes, I understand that your childhood traumas and abuse make relationships and connection dangerous. I hear you, out there on the margins, telling me that trust and vulnerability can get you killed.

For millions and millions of us, connecting with others is terrifying. And exposing. But it doesn't change the reality.

Loneliness is killing you.

It's killing me.

I don't think any of us set out to spend our days bowling alone[42] or otherwise hiding away from sunlight, laughter, petting the neighbor's dog, and developing relationships.

But here we are.

So from this point forward, internalize this:

Choosing to do life alone is choosing to die early.

Choosing to do life alone is choosing to have an anxious life.

And choosing to do life alone is a choice to take everyone around you down with you.

We must choose connection.

Because when we're lonely, especially when we're surrounded by people who love us, we slowly drown our loved ones. We hurt those trying to connect with us but who can't figure out how. Our family members who are wondering why we return our customers' calls late into the evening, but we don't say "I love you" at bedtime. Or our kids who are desperately wondering what is so damn amazing about that little shiny digital box that prevents you from looking them in the eye when they're talking.

And so your choice to be lonely isn't just a choice to slowly fade away.

Being lonely isn't a way to hide.

---

[42] Shout out to Robert Putnam and his ahead-of-its-time book *Bowling Alone: The Collapse and Revival of American Culture* (New York: Simon & Schuster, 2000).

It's a choice to be anxious, burned out, and electric.

The good news is, you can choose something different.

THE TRUTH ABOUT CONNECTIONS AND TECHNOLOGY

Yes, I hear the naysayers out there. You tell me about the amazing people you've met playing online video games, or how you stay connected to your friends through online chats, and how you're able to travel more because you can Face-Time with the kids and even FaceTime their first steps, soccer games, and recitals.

In our modern world, we can be connected with anyone, anywhere, at any time. We talk-to-text without taking our hands off the steering wheel, we can ask Alexa anything, AI (Artificial Intelligence) advancements are being developed at speeds beyond comprehension, and we will soon be able to know just about everything, all the time.

Every one of these things is true. We are the most digitally connected generation in the history of humankind. Yet all the data about skyrocketing loneliness, increases in diseases of despair, and the continual flattening-out (and even decline) in human life expectancy is also true. What's happening?

We suddenly exported all human interactions onto little boxes, onto mainframes, and into the cloud.[43] Our faces,

---

[43] I still have no idea what that is. It sounds like the Wizard of Oz or Harry Potter or something. I think it's just a bunch of servers

our jokes, our anger, our expressions, sadness, dreams, and pictures of our kids have been transferred into the Metaverse and memes. My friends call me a Luddite, but even I have found myself attending fewer sporting events, concerts, and having fewer hangouts at local pubs. Why go to a concert or football game and have some idiot spill beer on me when I can sit on my couch and take it all in on my 65-inch TV?[44]

I do love technology. I owe my life and my career to it.

I love not having to wait to hear about my wife's doctor's visit.

I love finding out in real time how my son did on his math test.

I love talking to my parents on the phone, sharing hilarious and wildly inappropriate memes with my friends, and being able to check the weather, the movies, or who won the fights wherever I happen to be.

It just all comes at a cost.

I can text my wife all day and tell her how much I love her, but she's only getting data. The little shiny box informs her that I love her—but she misses out on my body, my vocal tone, my actions, my energy, my posture, my warmth, my

---

in some massive warehouses, but I guess "server in a warehouse" doesn't have the same ring to it as "in the cloud."

[44] I don't actually have a 65-inch TV, but I often think it would be awesome if I did. And then I just read a book.

embrace, and me picking up my underwear. That's how she knows and feels love.

Communication is not connection.

Technology allows for communication, not connection.

Technology satisfies the data part of my brain: the *who*, *what*, *when*, *where*, and *how*. It doesn't allow the part of my brain and body that registers connection to be fully seen and experienced.

I only truly know who I am, and where I am, in relationship to those next to me. Technology leaves me over-informed and under-experienced. Folks know a lot of stuff about me, and I see a lot of things about them, but we don't know each other at all.

And here's where this has gone from bad to worse in just a few short years.

As a culture, we don't borrow things anymore. We don't ask for help anymore. We don't visit with our neighbors or reach out to our co-workers. We'd rather order sugar on Amazon delivery, or eggs on the grocery delivery app, than walk next door to ask for what we need. We'd rather Uber than request a ride to the airport from a friend. We'd rather spend money we don't have and put movers on the credit card than ask our buddies from church or work to give up their Saturday to help us load up the U-Haul.

We have apps that deliver flowers to our wives, that send subscription-style gifts to our husbands, complete with an AI-generated love note.

We are outsourcing community, connection, and, ultimately, love.

And practically overnight, we have pulled away from allowing others the gift of providing support or assistance. We are robbing our neighbors and friends from having a purpose or feeling needed or wanted, all because we don't want to bother or burden anyone.

Worse still, I believe other people's lives are made worse by my having needs. I sometimes find myself thinking others are worse off because I'm around.

If you get nothing else from this book, know this: You are not a burden.

And I'll say it one more time so you will read the words again, and hopefully tattoo this on your soul:

You are not a burden.

GETTING CONNECTED

Okay, you get it. We're lonely, withering on the vine, and our bodies are sounding the anxiety alarms.

So what do we do? How do we get connected and build a non-anxious life?

Many authors have written about the loneliness epidemic. In *Own Your Past, Change Your Future*, I wrote an entire chapter about making new friends, engaging with new friends, and ways to connect. I recommended making friendships a priority, looking for shared experiences, and going first to extend hospitality. I also suggested saying yes to invitations and adventures, getting out of your house to be where people are, and finding people to serve. All these efforts will set you on the path toward making new friends and connections.

But I think there's something underneath friendship that truly gets at the heart of loneliness. Something that burrows deep beneath our hearts, minds, and bodies, and ultimately plays a key role in a non-anxious life.

Yes, we have to make friends.

Yes, we have to invite people over, say yes, and take risks.

But beneath all the activities, we have to change our posture toward the world.

We have to choose love.

CHOOSING LOVE

Many of you just threw up in your mouth. I get it.

Love is blah. Gross. Lame. Soft.

Go ahead and roll your eyes. I did too.

Take your time . . . I'll wait.

Now that you're back, I want you to stamp this on your bones.
The foundation and core of a non-anxious life
is based on a single premise:
You are fully seen, heard, and known, and you are still loved.
And you fully know others and choose to love them too.

Love means someone (or a group of folks) knows everything about you, including your darkest thoughts, the worst things you've done, the horrible madness that has happened to you—

And they show up anyway.

And you for them.

To be fully known and fully loved: that is non-anxious living.

Love is the cornerstone.

Love is a posture of abundance.

Love isn't about possession, it's about open hands.

Love is a choice, made daily, to go second in times of plenty and to charge ahead first in times of danger.

As the great poet Steven Connell says, "Love is a promise that I will be right here."

Stephen Porges, a best-selling author and research scientist, reports: "Love, as a neurophysiological construct . . . provides a pair-bond to promote safety in a challenging environment."[45] The glue that holds us together is love.

I once asked a friend who was a member of an elite military unit if he and his comrades love one another when on mission. He responded, "A unique and indescribable love."

Without love, friends are buddies.

Spouses are roommates.

---

[45] Stephen W. Porges, *The Polyvagal Theory: Neurophysiological Foundations of Emotions, Attachment, Communication, Self-Regulation* (New York: W. W. Norton & Company, 2011), 185.

Neighbors are in the way.

Co-workers are trying to take what's rightfully yours.

When I was spun out and sizzling with anxiety, I was overwhelmed with information. I'd retreated into my own head and was consumed with thinking and solving, learning and knowing. My fists were clenched too tightly to be able to offer or receive love.

I was so locked in and locked up, it never occurred to me that I was worth being loved. By my wife, my son, or my friends.

And the alarms rang without ceasing.

I finally came to terms with reality: what I was doing wasn't working.

So I opened my hands and began learning how to let go.

I learned that love is showing up. And being there. And saying, "I do." And saying, "I will."

Love is consistent. Love is discipline—doing even when I don't want to.

I remember one time my friend Kevin and I were talking on the phone. He's super-wise, a tech executive with a deep heart for people on the margins of his community. Somebody I consider a close, brotherlike friend.

As we were getting off the phone, he said, "I love you."

And I was like, *Uh . . . nope.*

No.

To me, that *L*-word was reserved for my dog, my wife, and my kids . . . and occasionally my parents if one of them said it first. And Dorito tacos. And Gibson guitars.

I was most certainly not down with one of my friends telling me he loved me.

Now fast-forward 10 years, and rarely do my friends and I get off the phone without saying "I love you"—grown-ass men, some with massive salaries, others with massive bellies or muscles, depending on their addiction.

What changed for me?

I've done too many funerals and shown up to too many death scenes where people are gasping for air and a dream of one more moment with their loved one, just to tell them that they are loved.

Love doesn't mean soft. Love doesn't mean weak. Love doesn't mean powerless.

Love means you are strong enough to die in someone else's stead.

Love means you'll lay it all on the line.

You won't keep secrets. You'll tell the truth. You'll keep your covenants.

LOVE LOOKS LIKE . . .

Let me boldy state: If you don't have love, if you don't have friendship and connection and community, your anxiety alarms will ring off the wall.

Over time, everything will disintegrate to ash. Your marriage. Your business. Your relationship with your kids. Your neighborhood. Everything.

In the real world, love looks like . . .

- Treating customers with dignity.
- Doing excellent, honest good work at your job, even if it's not your passion or your dream job.
- Closing your laptop and putting down your phone every time your spouse or child walks into the room, even if only to look them in the eye and tell them, "Hey, let me finish sending this one message or email."

Love looks like . . .

- You never cheat or betray someone's trust.
- You choose the lower position and seek to meet your spouse's needs. And he or she does the same for you.
- You say, "I'm sorry." And "I forgive you."
- You love yourself enough to eat right, exercise, keep a gratitude journal, and see a counselor.
- You have people over. Stop making excuses, leave the laundry piled in the corner, and open up your door.
- You sleep with a shoe as your pillow on the floor of the ICU waiting room, praying that God will spare the life of your friend.

And I could go on and on.

Now let's just admit it:

Love is really hard. Choosing connection can be awful. Most of us don't have a good model for it.

And making new friends as an adult is the absolute worst. It's terrible. I'm a social guy and I hate it. My wife assures me that I'm *super*-awkward.

You've had people over who don't get the signals on when to leave, right? You stand up and they just keep sitting. You slap your knee and lean toward the door . . . and they pour another drink. Or you go upstairs and do the bedtime routine with your kids—baths, books, songs—and you come back down and you-know-who is STILL WATCHING TELEVISION!

Making friends is hard. Incredibly hard.

Love is one of the most difficult shifts to make, especially if you've been hurt or burned in the past.

But if you want to build a non-anxious life, you have to.

TACTILE TIPS FOR LOVE AND FRIENDSHIP

Here are a few important things to keep in mind as you begin to incorporate love and friendship into your life.

1) *Love and friendship are skills that you practice.* In *Own Your Past, Change Your Future*, I wrote: "This is about physiology, psychology, and spirituality. This is as complex as brain chemistry, hormone function, and gene expression. This is also as simple as someone bringing you tacos when you're grieving or helping you change a tire in your driveway."[46]

---

[46] John Delony, *Own Your Past, Change Your Future: A Not-So-Complicated Approach to Relationships, Mental Health, and Wellness*

We often hear words like *love* or *friendship* and we head for the hills. We over-dramatize them, we over-spiritualize them—basically, we make them much more difficult than they need to be.

From this point forward, think of love and friendship as skills. Things you will do.

- Show up.
- Lend a hand.
- Ask how someone's doing and actually pay attention to their answer.
- Be on time.
- Remember and honor the things that are important to the ones you love (birthdays, types of flowers, hobbies).
- Give generously of your most precious resource: your time.

You will mess this up.

You'll forget.

You'll be late.

You'll bring dessert with peanuts in it.

Or you'll arrive and not know anything about fixing air conditioners.

Keep practicing.

2) *Love and friendship are not about always having the right thing to say.* Often silence and presence are the most important.

(Franklin, TN: Ramsey Press, 2022), 169.

After my wife endured two tragic miscarriages, we were cautiously optimistic when we found out she was pregnant yet again. The pregnancy was moving along fine, under the care of a fantastic doctor, when my wife suffered a tubal rupture of an ectopic pregnancy. I was at work when she called me. I dropped everything, picked up our son as he was being let out of school, and raced over to the hospital.

Glimpsing the look in the OB-GYN's eyes as she took off running down the hall to rush my wife into emergency surgery, I had a horrifying thought: *This is the last time I will ever see my wife alive.*

I'd been to enough emergency situations in my career. I knew that look.

A friend came and picked up our son, and I headed to the waiting room by myself. I hadn't called anyone—I was shaken to my core and just trying to pull myself together. A little later, I looked up, and without fanfare, my great friend SJ was walking through the doors of the waiting room. He had shown up on his own.

He sat down next to me.

And he said nothing.

I didn't speak either.

We both sat on the floor of that waiting room in silence until the doctor came out to the waiting room some 45 minutes later.

She told me she had been unable to save the baby, but my wife was going to be okay.

As reality sank in, I melted against the chair.

SJ reached over and grabbed my shoe and gave it a light squeeze.

I looked over and he had tears streaming down his face.

My strong-but-kindhearted friend, a rancher and children's author, was crying tears for me that I was not yet able to cry.

And he never said a word.

When it comes to love and friendship, we often try and fill every space with jokes or opinions or unsolicited advice that we got from a framed photo in a church bathroom.

Don't.

Just show up. In times of tragedy or challenge, speak as little as possible, offer hugs or a hand to hold, keep your advice to yourself unless specifically asked—and do bring tacos or a casserole.

Your presence is enough.

3) *Friendship and love mean considering the needs of others before your own.* We have transformed love and human connection into a transactional exchange. We love people because of what we can get from them. We interact with others as a means of networking. This has thinned out connection and taken the soul from love and friendship. It has cheapened relationships and made the people in our lives a commodity, where it now seems every human exchange rests on an ugly premise: *What can this person do for me?*

When you love, you give. You seek to serve. Not because you're some kind of martyr, but because the highest honor is seeing to it that others feel appreciated and safe.

When you are a friend, you choose the backseat. You pick up the tab if you're able. You grill up something other than burgers if they're vegan, and you also don't cram your dietary choices down their throat. You lend a hand with their big chores: cleaning out the garage, reorganizing a closet, painting a room.

Sure, this idea of putting others' needs and preferences before your own can be abused. You can only truly love and be a good friend if you're well and whole. This means you have to take care of yourself. Running yourself into the ground just to impress and please others is not love or friendship. It is codependency.

Love is serving and meeting others' needs from a place of strength and joy, not desperation and approval-seeking.

As you do this, you'll naturally pull your gaze up from staring at your belly button to seeing the eyes of the loved ones and strangers standing right in front of you.

This is choosing connection.

This is the non-anxious life.

CLOSING THOUGHTS ON LOVE

We currently live in a culture that's brimming over with anger, worry, and chronic stress. Our cultural ethos is crushing, grinding busyness.

It's not working.

You can't rant or manipulate your way to peace and prosperity. It's a failed proposition.

You can't scream and rage your way to turn someone's opinion. No one has ever changed religions or recommitted themselves to a romantic relationship because they lost an argument.

But I do stand behind what my friend and pastor Ian Simkins says: "Whatever you think your hate is accomplishing, love can do better."

Love works.

The non-anxious person rejects loneliness. He or she chooses connection, even when it's hard.

You choose love over hate, friendships over disconnection, and awkwardness over networking.

This is an entry point toward a non-anxious life.

—————— CHOOSE CONNECTION ——————

Chapter Summary and Next Steps

Summary:

- To be well and have a full life, you must choose connection, relationships, and love.
- You cannot do life alone.
- Other people are your emergency fund for life. Hardships and emergencies *will* come knocking at your door. If you have no one to call or lean on in

times of trouble, your brain and body will never let you rest.

- Science proves that loneliness is killing us.
- Choosing to do life alone is choosing to die early.
- Choosing to do life alone is choosing to have an anxious life.
- And choosing to do life alone is a choice to take everyone around you down with you.

Things to Do:

- Make a list of your friends. Spend time with the list and ask yourself why these folks are your friends and how you show up for each other.
- Make a smaller list of your closest friends—those you would call in the middle of the night if you needed help with an emergency. Spend time with this list and ask yourself why these folks are your friends and how you show up for each other.
- Make a list of friends you have lost touch with. People you share connection with but no longer interact with. Why have you lost touch? Are they folks you should consider reconnecting with? Apologizing to? Accepting an apology from?
- This weekend, spend some time outside until you see one or more of your neighbors. **Say hello.** Introduce yourself.

- When the time is right, instead of jumping on the internet, consciously ask a neighbor for a favor, like, "Can I borrow some _____?" or "Hey, could you help me with this?"
- Call an old friend you haven't talked to in a while. Ask them questions about themselves just to catch up. Yes, it will be weird . . . but worth it.
- Apologize to someone.
- Accept an apology from someone and then invite them to go hang out.
- **Download 10 free *Questions for Humans* conversation starters from johndelony.com/resources.**
- Invite someone, a couple, or a whole family over for dinner. It doesn't have to be fancy.

Ask Yourself:

- Is there anyone (or more than one) who I fully trust? Why or why not?
- Reflect on this statement: *"You are fully seen, heard, and known, and you are still loved. And you fully know others and choose to love them too."*
- Who knows me better than anyone else in the world? Why?
- Who do I know better than anyone else in the world? Why?
- Why do I not let people get close to me?

- What are some ways I can start today to be more open to others?

Additional Resources:

- Go to johndelony.com/resources for a list of books, podcasts, and tools to help you start down the path toward a non-anxious life.

THE
6 DAILY CHOICES

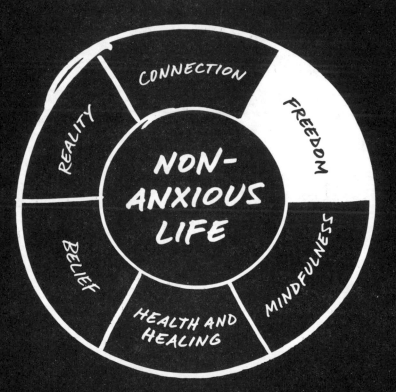

CHAPTER 6

CHOOSE FREEDOM

I didn't know how we were going to pay our bills.

I made a good salary. My wife made a great salary. We didn't take vacations, and we bought our headboard off Craigslist for $50. For some extra income, I taught additional college classes, took on writing or consulting gigs, and even accepted a secondary administrative assignment. But we still owed so much money. More than six figures in student loans. And we didn't own much of anything. A couple of old, unsightly vehicles and some used, cobbled-together furniture.

Yet we were coming up short. Every month.

And though we didn't buy furniture, cars, or vacations, I had a spending problem. I bought the stupidest things. Like multiple guitars and amplifiers. More supplements than my body could ever digest (I had the most expensive pee in the country). The t-shirts or shoes that best represented me. Expensive candles. Canvases to make my own terrible art. And I never got rid of anything; I just added more and more. I also didn't buy nice, quality things, so I ended up with junk I didn't really like that we would soon have to replace. So while I was patting myself on the back for not blowing money on expensive things . . . I was letting our family finances drip out of a hole in my wallet. Death—and debt—by a thousand cuts.

Since we usually couldn't afford much of anything, I maxed out every card we had. And when maxed, I'd just roll that balance to a higher-limit card. Sometimes I used my student loans as consolidation loans, moving debt from one pile to another. I was well versed in scheming, scrambling, and stealing from Peter to pay Paul.[47] Then, once a month, the bills would arrive, and I'd bathe in shame and make all kinds of promises about how I was a changed man. And I'd last about 36 hours in my new life before I was convinced I needed something else.

With all the extra jobs, I was also scheduled beyond the brink. My calendar was like a pair of skinny jeans at a Green Day reunion show: too much stuff crammed into too small of a container. I was constantly running from meeting to appointment to workout to budget review to MMA training to grad school to bedtime. And of course, I was late to everything.

I was late to church, work, grad school, and dates with my wife. I'd be late to kickboxing and jujitsu, then late getting home to bed.

---

[47] Maybe "Pay Paul" is where they got the name "Paypal"?

My body lived on a steady diet of cortisol and adrenaline, supplemented by my constant supply of yeses.

I said yes to everything because saying no felt like failing. Failing myself and everyone I was trying to please. I carried so much guilt and shame around having boundaries, I didn't have any. I convinced myself the world needed me.

Shame was a dragon always breathing at my neck. And if I stopped even briefly, it would catch me in its jaws, pin me down, and I'd be lost for a few days in a spiral of despair. So I kept running. I kept earning. I kept spending. I kept saying yes. I kept adding more and more crap.

I was slowly drowning in everything.

And I was the associate dean of students at a university.

My colleagues and students could feel how out-of-my-mind anxious I was. But my brain and body knew most of all: I was in danger. In danger of getting laid off, losing my house, and not being able to provide for my family.

Worst of all, my family and I had no freedom. The story I told myself was *This is all my fault.* I had not kept us safe. I had driven us into a ditch with my foot hammered on the gas, and now we were stuck, spinning our wheels but going nowhere. I was just digging a deeper and deeper hole.

Someone who's oppressed, trapped, chained up, or unable to make decisions for and about their future will be anxious. It was here I decided, finally, that I wanted something different for us. A better life. From the depths of the ditch, I decided to choose freedom.

That's the next daily choice: *Choose Freedom.*

FOUR AREAS FOR FREEDOM

When I say choose freedom, I'm not being flippant. I know there are billions of people across the globe who are not free from political, cultural, and religious oppression. I know there are untold numbers of people in the United States who are being trafficked, persecuted, and marginalized. I understand this—and I humbly acknowledge how unqualified I am to speak on most of these matters. Not wanting to add to the noise, I defer to the experience and wisdom of the experts on these important global topics.

The freedom I'm talking about is much more local. I'm referring to both the conscious and unconscious ways we give away our lives in exchange for the promise of the good life. In other words, where we trade our freedom for illusions.

Most people, most of the time, are living their lives for other people. To challenge you to choose freedom is my way of urging all of us to consciously put ourselves back in the driver's seat of our own life.

In this chapter, I've intentionally chosen to focus on four themes related to freedom. These themes have repeatedly surfaced as I've dug into the anxiety literature, talked with thousands of people, and struggled for freedom in my own life. As we discuss these four themes in detail, do your best to deeply internalize where you are, right now, and what it would feel like to experience freedom in each particular area. It's easy to roll your eyes without digging in.

Don't.

You're worth being free.

Money

I recently took a heartbreaking call on *The Ramsey Show* from a man who was drowning in consumer and student loan debt. Through a series of misfortunes—a medical issue, corporate downsizing, and his own poor decisions—he was in a dark hole and didn't see a way out.

He was so tired of getting hassled by creditors, so angry writing checks each month for long-ago purchases, and so discouraged by his predicament, he was considering taking his life. He was done.

Chances are, if you've found yourself buried under a pile of debt, you probably feel done too.

Solving for freedom with money means you don't owe anyone anything.

Read that again.

You don't owe anyone anything.

If you're not debt-free (including your house, vehicles, etc.)—I want you to close your eyes and pretend you don't owe any person or business any money. Feel it. Imagine if you got to keep your entire paycheck every month, minus a few utility bills, insurance, and property taxes. What if all your money, beyond what the government requires, was yours to keep?

Imagine laughing when your abusive, crooked boss tells you to stay late one too many times. Imagine saying, "No, thank you," and just gathering your things and walking out the door.

Imagine calmly calling the HVAC company when your air conditioner breaks instead of having a panic attack.

Imagine the joy of being able to buy clothes for the family at church who lost their house in a fire. Or picking up the tab of the clearly exhausted dad with three bonkers kids sitting next to you at Waffle House. Imagine just giving a neighbor your old truck. Or helping a friend's kid go to college. Or digging a well in another country for people who don't have clean water.

This is freedom.

You get to decide what you do with your life.

When you owe people money, you don't get to decide what you do tomorrow. The bank does. Your father-in-law does. The department store does.

When you owe people money, you spend your hours working to pay for things you've already purchased. You help other people get wealthy and live the life *they* want to live instead of creating safety in your own life and in the life of your family.

And before you jump in, I don't want to hear your arguments about financial margins, debt ratios, or any other economic theories you've devised, like a toddler, to get whatever you want, whenever you want it, by any means necessary. Look around! Your Instagram-informed, get-rich schemes aren't working.

We're broke.

We're enslaved.

As a country, as a culture, and as individual households, we've written checks we will never be able to cash. Government leaders spend your money in ways they would NEVER spend their personal funds.

To illustrate, if we were to convert the size and scope of the debt of the United States,[48] it would look like this:

- Your take-home salary would be $67,521 per year.
- You would spend $113,820 per year, putting $46,299 on your credit card.
- While you were recklessly spending like this, you would also already have $474,282 in existing credit card debt.
- And you would keep doing this, over and over again, year after year.

The picture in our own homes isn't all that much better. According to research from Ramsey Solutions, the average person in America struggles with debt—and over half (59 percent) of Americans said they worry about their general finances. Thirty-seven percent of Americans are either struggling or in crisis when it comes to their money. Just under half (45 percent) said they have at least $1,000 in savings while 19 percent have less than $1,000 in savings—and over a third (36 percent) have no savings at all.[49]

We're in a perpetual state of paying for last month's food, and last summer's concerts, and last year's medical bills with next month's dollars.

---

[48] "U.S. Budget vs. Family Budget," Federal Budget in Pictures, https://www.federalbudgetinpictures.com/us-budget-vs-family-budget/.
[49] "The State of Personal Finance," Ramsey Solutions (October 2022).

The thinking part of your brain can rationalize your "good deal." Your 0 percent down. Your magical interest rate. Or those leather seats.

Your rational brain can say, "I deserve it" and "YOLO!" But the part of your brain designed to warn you of impending dangers is sounding the alarms.

Your body is anxious for a reason. You are one accident or illness or job loss away from the whole house of cards coming down.

Freedom with money is not owing anyone. Ever. Regardless of how good the deal is. This freedom allows you to enjoy purchases like cars and nice things, without the anxiety. This freedom also allows you to be generous and care for people beyond comprehension. It's being able to make a difference for the causes you care about.

My friend Dave Ramsey calls it financial peace.

I call it freedom.

Clutter and Stuff

Our entire way of life is built on the concept of growth. We are taught from a young age to "Go get . . ." To make, create, and earn. We're encouraged to collect experiences, date different people, and update our clothes (there are even subscriptions now!). We get new makeup, haircuts, shoes, and hobbies. Within a few months of buying a new home or a new car, we are already thinking about the makeover. Or the upgrade.

Culturally, we shop as a way to relieve tension. We buy the right watch, the right jacket, and the right shoes to demonstrate our worth to other people. We watch the right shows, we buy the right books, we collect the right things. And thanks to social media, we're no longer just keeping up with the Joneses, but we're keeping up with every single person on the planet.

In all fairness, our brains have evolved across countless centuries for times of scarcity. For life and death. We are wired to collect and consume. We're also recent descendants of a generation that lived through the Great Depression. My granddad straightened nails to reuse them—because he had to. He bought a two-bedroom, 800-square-foot house where he and my grandmother raised four kids. At the same time. Without murdering each other.[50]

My grandmother patched up jeans and handed them down to all her kids. And when the jeans simply didn't function as pants anymore, they were converted to blankets and quilts. Old quilts went from bedroom use, to couch use, to outdoor use, to blankets for the dogs. And when they were tattered and worn, they were washed and the threads were pulled to be used again.

My grandparents' generation kept everything. They saved every bolt, metal spring, and piece of wood because they simply couldn't afford more. And when their kids (our parents)

---

[50] My wife and I have much more space and I'm fairly certain she thinks about ending my life with some regularity. My granddad was truly part of the Greatest Generation.

discovered credit cards and HELOC loans, that next generation went the opposite direction: They set out to buy new things. Always new and shinier things.

Since then, consumption has become the name of the game. We have bought and consumed and stored. For decades.

And now we're being suffocated by our stuff.

As a culture, we've learned how to amass. But we have not learned the skills of removal. Of letting things go. We have no psychological construct for *enough*.

This is another way we've created a world that our brains and bodies cannot live in.

I was recently in Minnesota, hanging out with my friend Dawn Madsen. Her professional moniker is "The Minimal Mom," and through her podcast and other resources, she helps families shed clutter and chaos from their lives. While we were together, she introduced me to Fumio Sasaki and a concept called "The Silent To-Do List." In her *Declutter Your Home in 15 Minutes a Day* workbook, Dawn writes, "[Sasaki] says that every single material item in your house is sending out a message of something to do, and this message gets added to your to-do list without you knowing it!" Dawn adds, "Dishes stacked up by the sink say, 'Wash me, dry me, and put me away. Why can't you keep up with me?'" Or: "Laundry on the floor exclaims, 'Pick me up, put me in the laundry room, wash me, take care of me, put me away.'"[51]

---

[51] Dawn Madsen, *Declutter Your Home in 15 Minutes a Day: A Workbook Guiding You Through Each Room in Your House,* https://

Right now, I'm sitting in a corner of my basement, where I've carved out a little writing/reading/guitar jamming space. And if I look up from my laptop screen, I'm met by countless objects screaming at me. Guitars and amps and pedals yelling, "WHY AREN'T YOU PLAYING ME? What happens if your favorite punk band calls and YOU'RE NOT READY?!"

Hundreds of books shouting, "READ ME! READ ME AGAIN! Do you want to be dumb? You'll never be as smart as Drs. Huberman or Attia or Norton if you don't stop type-type-typing and START READING!"

Old CDs (yes, I still have a bunch of them) begging me to play them.[52] Workout gadgets imploring me to get in better shape. A cheap air-hockey table asking me why I won't play with my son. Do I not love him? Am I too busy for him?

And that's just in this little room.

Madsen and Sasaki nailed it. Our stuff screams at us. It's relentless. Clutter and excessive consumption are directly linked to anxiety.

Obtaining material possessions also takes your most precious resource: your time. Every purchase costs you a piece of your life. My good friends Joshua Fields Millburn and Ryan Nicodemus, best-selling authors and founders of The

---

www.theminimalmom.com/workbook, 85.

[52] My everyday commute is like a scene from *The Matrix*, except I'm not dodging bullets; I'm dodging CDs flying all over the place. If this book sells enough copies, I'm going to finally get rid of the CD player in my truck. It's time.

Minimalists, say, "Every time you part with a dollar, you part with a tiny piece of your freedom. If you earn $20 an hour, then that $4 cup of coffee just cost you twelve minutes, that $800 iPad cost you a week, and that $40,000 new car cost you an entire year of freedom."[53]

Your stuff takes your money, your time, and your sanity. You feel responsible for your stuff. The feeling of *I need to do something about it* never goes away. Neither does the stuff. It's crammed in closets, jam-packed garages, under beds, and in storage units across your city.

Your storage spaces aren't just filled up with boxes and bicycles and VHS tapes and abandoned sports equipment. They're filled up with your memories. And time. We attach meaning and power to the things we own. To pieces of paper or fabric. We trap grandparents in antique furniture and past boyfriends in photographs.

Oh, and the emergency stash! We're always planning for the next emergency. We can't get rid of that old sweater 'cause what if the temperature drops to 30-below and the heater breaks and I need this gnarly thing as a seventh layer? Be honest: Do you still have the cake plate you got for your wedding? You never use cake plates, but you keep it because Aunt Cathy bought it and she may come over one day and start cranking out cakes!

---

[53] Joshua Fields Millburn and Ryan Nicodemus, *Love People/Use Things: Because the Opposite Never Works* (New York: Celadon, 2021), 63.

We have to stop.

Anxiety is worrying about the future in the present—and buying and cluttering things helps us pretend like we're hedging against future disasters.

Anxiety is trying to remain connected to people and memories and our histories through piles of artwork, old collections, and things someone else used to own.

Anxiety is the fantasy of *one day*. One day we'll get around to all those books. One day we'll eat those jars of pasta sauce no one likes. One day we'll start changing our own car oil or quilting like our great-grandmothers.

And so we buy another storage space. We pile stuff on top of stuff. We buy another organizing book or watch another home-improvement show on HGTV. Meanwhile, our anxiety alarms are ringing off the ceiling because we're suffocating, straitjacketed by all the stuff.

Recently I was going through a closet full of old clothes I hadn't worn in years. I came upon an old tweed jacket of my granddad's. He passed away several years ago, and I miss him dearly. I had not put that jacket on in almost a decade—it never fit me because I'm a bigger guy than he was. Still, I'd kept that jacket.

As I moved it over to the Keep pile yet again, this time I stopped. I took a deep breath as I held the piece of clothing and said out loud, "My granddad is not in this old jacket." I put my fist on my heart and said out loud, "He's in here.

"Gosh, I miss you, Granddad."

And I smiled.

And I got choked up a bit.

And I put the jacket in the Donate pile.

Time

I have a love/hate relationship with time. And by *love*, I mean I LOVE how much I HATE time. I honestly think I experience it differently than other people.

Time is a burden to me. There's never enough. It's always slipping away. Always keeping me from all the things I want to do. Always getting me into trouble.

But that's not really true. In his book *The Ruthless Elimination of Hurry*, theologian and best-selling author John Mark Comer says, "Our *time* is our life, and our attention is the doorway to our hearts."[54]

Time isn't this monster that is always trying to embarrass me at my workplace, cut short my hours with loved ones, or ruin my fun. Time isn't the problem.

My relationship to time is the problem. I disrespect time, yet it doesn't care. It continues to march on, *tick-tock, tick-tock*. I ignore time. I try to stretch time. I try to pretend it's not real.

And it keeps on ticking.

---

[54] John Mark Comer, *The Ruthless Elimination of Hurry: How to Stay Emotionally Healthy and Spiritually Alive in the Chaos of the Modern World* (Colorado Springs: Waterbrook, 2019), 234.

If you look at your calendar, I would bet money that most of you are just like me.

We can play all sorts of games with time and tell ourselves it doesn't matter, or that life will go on forever.

But every sunset brings us one day closer to our last day. Every heartbeat brings us closer to our final breath.

Time is a constant reminder that I'll never get it all done. That one day, my kids will have to ask someone else for their advice. Someone else will be in my job.

Time is a constraint I cannot escape with more money, more power, more muscles, more beauty, or more organization. So I try to cram it all in.

I've let my life become so chaotic, there is not a single minute in my day when I couldn't be—or shouldn't be—doing something else. I've loaded up my calendar with dates and speaking gigs and deadlines. I've got radio shows and media hits and work events and friend events. We have a vacation scheduled for a year from now, I know what time I'll be recording my show this time next year, and I've scheduled my morning routines down to the minute . . . There are no moments for me to unwind. Or think. Or let spontaneous adventures happen.

Want to know why your brain spins through hundreds of thoughts, especially focusing on the catastrophic, scary, and disorienting ones, just as you lay your head down on the pillow to go to sleep? Because that's the first sliver of space you've provided for it to do its most sacred activity: think.

Our bodies are screaming at us that we have too much

going on. That we must create space in our lives. That we need time to be bored, to process, to create, and to be with the ones we love.

Boundaries

A discussion on boundaries is worthy of its own book,[55] so I'll be brief and direct in my explanation.

Modern-day relationships can often be characterized as selfish, dysfunctional madness. *New York Times* best-selling author David Brooks acknowledges we live in a sick, insane culture "in which the needs of the self take priority over all other needs. The purpose of life is to self-actualize, to express your own autonomy and individuality."[56] He goes on to say,

> A healthy community is a thick system of rela-
> tionships. It is irregular, dynamic, organic, and
> personal. . . . People are up in one another's busi-
> ness, know each other's secrets, walk with each
> other in times of grief, and celebrate together in
> times of joy. . . . People help raise one another's

---

[55] Two incredible books on boundaries already exist: *Boundaries* by Drs. Henry Cloud and John Townsend, and *Set Boundaries, Find Peace* by Nedra Tawwab. I highly recommend them both.
[56] David Brooks, *The Second Mountain: The Quest for a Moral Life* (New York: Random House, 2019), 142.

kids. In these kinds of communities, which were typical in all human history until the last sixty years or so, people extended to neighbors the sorts of devotion that today we extend only to family. . . . The social pressure can be slightly overbearing, the intrusiveness sometimes hard to bear, but the discomfort is worth it because the care and benefits are so great.[57]

We discussed this need for love, friendship, and connection in chapter 5. We can no longer live lonely, isolated lives, staring down a telescope pointed at our own belly buttons.

But . . .

We have become a society free and clear of all boundaries. With the creation of the internet, email, social media, and smart phones, no one knows where they stop or other people start anymore. And because we don't know, we find ourselves living other people's lives. Or the way we think they expect us to live.

We say yes to things because we're scared of saying no. We sacrifice our health, our closest relationships, and our own sanity to try and show the world how great we are.

We're not empowered to rest, we do holidays the way the in-laws want them done, we take jobs to make other people proud, and we're shamed into accepting invitations.

---

[57] Brooks, *The Second Mountain*, 266–67.

We're peacekeepers, making sure everyone else is taken care of before we bother to ask ourselves how we're doing or what we need.

It's exhausting.

Best-selling authors Dr. Henry Cloud and Dr. John Townsend suggest we need boundaries because "[boundaries] define us. They define what is me and what is not me. A boundary shows me where I end and someone else begins, leading me to a sense of ownership. Knowing what I am to own and take responsibility for gives me freedom."[58]

In a recent episode of her *Unlocking Us* podcast, Dr. Brené Brown was discussing the unique relationship between compassion and boundaries. Turns out they are intimately linked.

During the podcast, Dr. Brown's sister Ashley said, "Boundaries come from believing in your time and your space enough to protect it."[59] *Bull's-eye.*

This means you take responsibility for saying, clearly, what you need. Love people enough to not force them to be mind readers. Own the things that bring you joy. Only then can you be of greatest value to the rest of the world.

---

[58] Henry Cloud and John Townsend, *Boundaries: When to Say YES, When to Say NO, to Take Control of Your Life* (Grand Rapids, MI: Zondervan, 1992), 31.

[59] Brené Brown, interview with Ashley Brown Ruiz, "Living BIG, Part 1 of 2", *Unlocking Us* podcast (December 28, 2022), https://brenebrown.com/podcast/living-big-part-1-of-2/.

Setting limits and boundaries is a way we can finally be free to do the messy work of connecting through love and friendship. Limits and boundaries let our bodies know where we are in time and space, and they give us room to make sure our needs are met.

When you start implementing boundaries, it will be hard on you and those around you. Some people will hate your boundaries.

New York Times best-selling author and licensed therapist Nedra Tawwab says,

> The hardest thing about implementing boundaries is accepting that some people won't like, understand, or agree with yours. Once you grow beyond pleasing others, setting your standards becomes easier. Not being liked by everyone is a small consequence when you consider the overall reward of healthier relationships.[60]

We can only have the messy, chaotic, deeply intertwined communities that David Brooks spoke of if we have purposeful and intentional boundaries. This is where the paradox of both deep, loving relationships and strong relational boundaries flow from separate streams into a single unified river. Only when I know who I am, what I am about, what my needs are, what my values are, and how I like to be treated

---

[60] Nedra Glover Tawwab, *Set Boundaries, Find Peace: A Guide to Reclaiming Yourself* (New York: TarcherPerigee, 2021), 61.

am I free to deeply engage in extraordinary connections and opportunities.

Our boundaries give us the chance to show up as our best for those who need us most. In a broken, splintering world, boundaries help us show up whole. When we clearly communicate our boundaries to others, we are giving them the opportunity to help meet our needs, to align (or not) with our values, and to have a clear sense of the potential connectivity and depth of their relationship with us.

As my friend Will Guidara, a world-class restaurateur and best-selling author, tells his waitstaff: "You can't fill up a patron's glass if your pitcher is empty." You have to take the time to fill up your pitcher so you can be about filling up other people's glasses.

You can't give what you don't have. You're not going to be compassionate and generous from an empty place.

And more importantly, if you can't be compassionate to yourself, you cannot be compassionate to others.

Boundaries are how you begin to make long-term investments in yourself and, ultimately, in and for others. Whether they're big boundaries or little boundaries, you have to be the champion of your time, talents, and resources.

Having boundaries around those three areas—your time, energy, and talents—is one of the most compassionate, responsible, loving things you can do.

Boundaries equal compassion. For you and for everyone else.

Boundaries give us freedom.

CHOOSING FREEDOM IN THE REAL WORLD

We are ready to begin to design and build a life with more freedom, margin, and space. Margin in your financial life, clutter-free spaces in your home, room in your calendar, and boundaries in your relationships.

In the section below, I have detailed some ways I've been able to find success in my day-to-day life in each of the four areas, and how countless others have reduced or eliminated anxiety for themselves too.

Start with Identity

First, we start with our new identity.

This idea comes from best-selling author James Clear, and it has been transformative in my life. If you read this chapter, get all fired up, and then throw everything away, cancel everything on your calendar, cut up your credit cards and quit spending money, and call your mother-in-law and yell into the phone, "NEVER AGAIN!" . . . it will be a disaster.

Why?

Because no matter what you throw away, however you pay off your debts, and however strong your boundaries are, **you** **will always go with you**. And since your body is always solving for what it knows, the same margin and space and debt issues will return in short order.[61]

---

[61] Make sure to check out *Atomic Habits* by James Clear. I highly recommend this book.

So instead of beginning with a bunch of goals and finish lines, we will begin with identity. Who are you? Who are you going to become?

In this new season, we are people who are *free*. We choose to live lives that are free from other people controlling, dictating, and driving us.

Say it out loud, right now.[62] "I am a person who is FREE! I am a person who chooses FREEDOM!"

So what does that mean across these four areas?

MONEY

I am a person who chooses freedom. I am a person who wants to live and give like I want to. So,

1. I will never borrow money again.[63]

   Ever.

   I will not be owned by any other person or financial institution.

2. If I am currently in debt, I will write down on a piece of paper every single dollar I owe someone else. Every debt including student loans, family or personal loans, credit cards, car loans (or leases), medical

---

[62] Of course, if you're in a library or an airport, you may want to whisper. Or maybe not. Go for it!

[63] Except, possibly, on a mortgage—see Dave Ramsey's *The Total Money Makeover: A Proven Plan for Financial Fitness* (Nashville: Thomas Nelson, 2009) for more specifics.

bills, store credit charges, and on and on. Write them all down and get a final number.

3. I will utilize Ramsey Solutions' Baby Steps method of paying off the debt in the quickest and most proven way possible. Since I am an adult, I will not expect my parents to keep paying off my debts, I will not wait on the government to come save me with money it has borrowed from taxpayers, and I will delay gratification and save up for things I want to buy.

    With cash.

4. I will establish a cash emergency fund as a way to peacefully, and immediately, deal with life's curve-balls. Because the dishwasher will break, your son will sprain his foot, or Covid. Remember Covid?

5. I will invest, save, and take care of my future self, making that a priority.

TIME

I am a person who chooses freedom. I am a person who wants to live and give like I want to. So, I will look at time as my single most precious asset.

1. I will take an inventory of my family's calendar. All our activities. I will allot each person a single activity per week. A single night out per week.

2. I will take inventory of how I use time. I will check my computer and cell phone logs and my social

media accounts for how much time I spend each day, week, month, and year on screens.

3. I will structure my day so that in almost every situation imaginable, I am on time, able to drive the speed limit, and arriving at meals, meetings, and events with grace and peaceful energy.

4. I will be prepared, engaged, and unhurried. Being busy will no longer be a way I show the world how important I am.

5. I will connect with somebody who will hold me accountable to keeping spaces open on my calendar.

CLUTTER AND STUFF

I am a person who chooses freedom. I am a person who wants to live and give like I want to. So, I will not surround myself with chaotic or clutter-filled environments. I also understand that if I have challenges with hoarding or addiction, accomplishing this might require professional intervention. But I am a person who is worth living a non-anxious life.

1. I am a person who puts effort into relationships and not into objects.

2. I am a person who does not evaluate myself based on what I do or do not own. Brand labels do not impress me or empower me.

3. Each day I will do something to organize myself for at least 10 minutes. This might mean deleting photos

or old text messages, paring down makeup or toiletries, or giving away junk in the garage.

a. I will get rid of clothes that don't fit or that I don't wear regularly. I will simplify my wardrobe and begin asking hard questions about brand labels and my self-worth.

b. I will throw away all trash and trinkets, and donate any and all items possible that might truly be of use or value to someone else.

The Basics of Decluttering Your Home

1. I will clean up my environment.
    a. Car a mess?
    b. Piles of laundry and junk?
    c. Kid toys and pet stuff everywhere?
2. I will look at my digital clutter.
    a. How many digital accounts do I have? Are my passwords for these accounts organized in one secure place?
    b. Can I cut subscriptions, unsubscribe from emails, etc.?
    c. Are my desktop icons a disaster?
3. I will declutter my brain, body, and spirit.
    a. Keep a journal on a regular basis. Write down what you feel, your successes, your challenges, your fears, and your aspirations. This is a place for

you to have an honest conversation with yourself that is outside your head.

b. Over time, use your journal to keep an inventory of your thoughts (especially the things you ruminate and obsess over). Write down the lightning-bolt thoughts: the ones that tell you you're a terrible father, the horrible memories, or your future worries. Challenge them for accuracy, truth, and reality.

BOUNDARIES

I am a person who chooses freedom. I want to be in deep, intertwined, and supportive relationships. And in order to do that, I have strong, firm, and committed boundaries for my mind, boundaries for my rest and activity, boundaries for my needs and desires, boundaries for my relationships, and boundaries for my work.

1. I will not subject myself to a dangerous, poison-filled work environment. A job that is challenging and uncomfortable is different than being regularly abused, disrespected, undervalued, or taken advantage of. The work should push me farther than I think I'm able to go. My leaders should be supportive, caring, respectful with wages, and provide me with the resources to accomplish my job. Otherwise, I will research and apply for other options.

2. I will begin to ask very difficult questions and make concrete decisions.
   a. What do I need to be well?
   b. What—and who—drains me, and who should I spend less/no more time with?
   c. Who should I spend more time with?
   d. When I think of people I do not like being around, what characteristics do they have in common?
   e. What gives me relational harmony? Who challenges me and also deeply cares for me? Who is using me like a vampire and I'm allowing it to continue?
3. Which people bring me peace? What work brings me peace? Of course, peace doesn't mean a kicked-back, easy life free of struggle, disagreements, or heartache. But during the challenging times, who and what brings me peace?
   a. What do I need to remove from my life so I can make this a reality?
4. I will be a person who *never* yells. Not at my kids, not at other adults, not at other people's kids, and not at unsuspecting drivers on the highway. I am a person with self-control over my emotions, my reactions, and the words and energy I put into the world.
5. I am a person who does not tolerate abuse, gossip, or evil-spirited interactions. I will simply remove myself from these situations. Or seek to have the abusers or aggressors removed. I will not look for

fights, and the number of hills I am willing to die on are few and very far between. I will be able and willing to fight but will choose not to in almost every situation.

--------------- **CHOOSE FREEDOM** ---------------

Chapter Summary and Next Steps

Summary:

- If you are not free, your body knows you are not safe.
- When your body feels it is not safe, it will sound the alarms.
- If you owe people money, regardless of how good the interest rate or payment plan is, your body knows someone else can take away your home, your transportation, your food, healthcare, and more. And your body will sound the alarms.
- If you are surrounded by chaos and clutter, your mind and body become overwhelmed by ongoing engagement with "stuff." In turn, your body will sound the alarms.
- If you have no margin on your calendar, you are not safe. If you are trying to be all things to all people, letting your child's activities, your hobbies, or your lack of discipline wreck your calendar, your body will be stressed and anxious.

- If you have weak or no relational boundaries, if other people have more voice in your life than you do, your body will never feel safe.

Things to Do:

- **Resolve to pay off all your debts.** Go to johndelony .com/resources to get connected to Financial Peace University, the best program in the world for getting out of debt.
- Take an inventory of your stuff, from your garages, closets, storage units, barns, and sheds to what's under the beds, in drawers, and on your bookshelves. Be honest about the chaos and clutter in your physical environment. What can you sell or give away RIGHT NOW that would make your life more peaceful and less cluttered?
- Take an inventory of your digital chaos and clutter. Passwords, subscriptions, accounts, email accounts, business email lists, endless hard drives of pictures and videos. Begin deleting, unsubscribing, and canceling.
- Take a hard look at your calendar. First weekly, then monthly, then annual. Wipe off the calendar and start from scratch. Begin with important items like connection, family time, exercise and restorative practices, and mandatory things such as work and school. Then, slowly—and with extreme intentionality—add back things like after-school

activities, church activities, civic and community responsibilities, and so forth. Make sure you build in margin.

- Make a list of who directs your life. It could be a spouse, a boss, or your mother-in-law. On most days, who is telling you what to do and how to do it?

Ask Yourself:

- Writing down *every single debt*, in order of smallest to largest, how much money do I owe?
- What is my relationship with money? Do I love it? Chase it? Hate it? Hide from it?
- Am I willing to be uncomfortable for one to three years, drive used cars, not go out, and buy little of anything for the chance to be free forever?
- What is my relationship to my stuff? This includes collections, clothes, gifts, storage spaces, furniture, and so on. Why do I struggle to get rid of things I don't need, don't use, or don't even want?
- How over-filled and over-stressed is my calendar? Am I trying to do too much with not enough in order to feel worth or importance? Do I feel compelled to say yes to anyone who needs my help or expertise? Where does that come from?
- Why is it hard for me to create and hold firm boundaries? Do I struggle with telling family members no, or being abused by toxic work or romantic

relationships? What small boundaries can I start to put into practice?

Additional Resources:

- Go to johndelony.com/resources for a list of books, podcasts, and tools to help you start down the path toward a non-anxious life.

THE 6 DAILY CHOICES

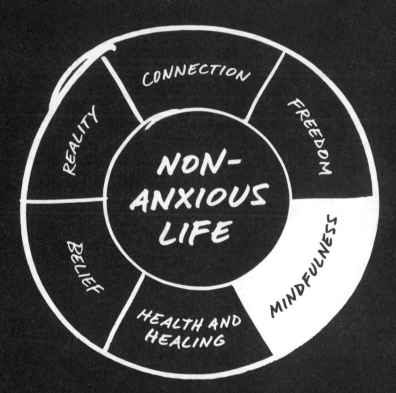

CONNECTION

FREEDOM

REALITY

NON-ANXIOUS LIFE

MINDFULNESS

BELIEF

HEALTH AND HEALING

CHAPTER 7

CHOOSE MINDFULNESS

A few years ago, I was putting my shoes on to head to the gym. It was well before 5:30 in the morning, and the world outside was quiet and dark. Suddenly, without warning, my five-year-old daughter just appeared standing next to me. It was like she silently manifested herself from bed to living room, as young kids are weirdly able to do.

My wife was up and made my daughter some oatmeal while I continued to get ready. Grabbing my watch and headphones, I made my way through the kitchen. As I passed my daughter, who by now was quietly coloring in the early-morning vapor between awake and asleep, I leaned over and gently kissed her on top of her tiny little head and whispered, "Good morning, baby. I love you."

Instantly my daughter became enraged and began flailing her mop of blonde hair about.

"*Woahhh!*" I said.

She interrupted me, ripping at full volume: "I wish you never existed!"

My wife popped up over the table, in defense of me. She said, "No, ma'am! In this house, we treat each other with dignity and respect. We do not talk to each other that way!"

My daughter responded with an impudent, powerful voice, "All he ever says is 'I love you,' and 'You're so brilliant,' and 'You're so beautiful and gritty and strong' . . ." She followed up with her final declaration, practically ripped from the pages of a Twisted Sister lyric, "I've had it, I can't take this, and I'm not going to live like this anymore!"

I looked at my wife, forced a crooked smile, and said, "I've had a lot of grad school, but I never took *that* class." And with that, I headed out the front door.

Closing the door behind me, I took two steps outside and stopped. The first thought that popped into my mind was *Yep. Maybe if you were home more and not always on the road, she'd want you around. Maybe if you cared about her more than your stupid writing career, she'd want hugs instead of distance.*

And then the kicker:

I suck at being a dad.

THE INNER VOICE

I despise the inner voice. Or if you're like me, voices—plural.

You know, that silent voice only you can hear. The voice that never shuts up. Always whispering. Always judging. Always complaining. Always clamoring for attention. Always getting in the way, yet somehow sounding helpful.

The inner voice likes to talk about other people's faults *and* my faults, simultaneously propping me up and tearing me down. Lying, blaming, coercing. Telling me how worthless and stupid and unattractive I am. Making excuses, starting imaginary fights, and constantly stoking the fire.

My inner voice never shuts up.

Building a non-anxious life involves taking on all the voices in your head—whether yours, your dad's, an old lover's, or a coach from high school. It involves challenging them when appropriate, creating distance between you and the babble, and learning not to believe every thought you think. This is about choosing peace inside your own mind.

We must *Choose Mindfulness.*

For real. I know. My eyes rolled out the back of my head too. Mindfulness makes me think of some bearded guy sitting on a cloud, or a woman in light-blue spandex sitting on a pillow in the middle of a forest, acting dramatic and serious about doing nothing.

This is not what I'm talking about.

I'm talking about the energetic core, pulsing beneath the idea of *control what you can control.* I often tell people to shift their focus from what they are fired-up and angry about and can't change, to the few things in the world they can control.

They understandably get annoyed and say, "Oh, that's cute. How do I do that?"

My answer?

Mindfulness.

And as shown through some incredible work by Dr. Jud Brewer, mindfulness is a powerful intervention for silencing the anxiety alarms.

WHAT IS MINDFULNESS?

Let's begin with a definition by landmark mindfulness researcher and Harvard psychology and medical school professor Dr. Ellen Langer. She writes,

> Just as mindlessness is the rigid reliance on old categories, mindfulness means the continual creation of new ones. Categorizing and recategorizing, labeling and relabeling as one masters the world. . . . [This is] an adaptive and inevitable part of surviving in the world.[64]

Say you were to look at a photograph of a raging river. Everything in the photo is beautiful, still, and contained. Now imagine you got in a helicopter and flew to the banks of the river in the exact location of the photograph. The water would not be a captured, frozen image. It would be alive, moving, and dragging chunks of rock and mud, changing the landscape as it flowed.

When it comes to our thoughts and how we experience the world, our mind wants to capture the raging rivers of our lives in still photos so it can categorize them as either friend

---

[64] Ellen J. Langer, *Mindfulness* (Boston: Da Capo Press, 1989), 63.

or foe, dangerous or safe—and then decide which photo album to put them in. This worked when the world was a much simpler, quieter place. But old categories and boxes no longer serve our modern world. It's hard to capture much of anything when it's all moving so fast.

Mindfulness, as Dr. Langer points out, is teaching our brain a different way of learning and living and experiencing the world. She suggests that mindfulness is about no longer staring at the picture, but instead, experiencing the raging river. And rather than trying to label and capture the river for the purpose of filing it, judging it, and measuring it, we must take notice of its new shapes, its new directions, and the different challenges that lie ahead. Neuro-researcher, professor, and best-selling author Dr. Dan Siegel says this new way of thinking and seeing the world actually alters the structure of your brain.

Don't miss this: Mindfulness is work—because you're growing new parts of your brain.[65] You can learn to hold things loosely. Open your hands. And begin interacting with the world in new ways, by new patterns, and with new understanding. This also plays a key role in learning to change the way you talk to yourself and others, transforming your life from one of mindless reaction to being intentionally proactive.

---

[65] Daniel J. Siegel, *Mindsight: The New Science of Personal Transformation* (New York: Bantam Books, 2010), 5, 277.

Here's an example. Say you and your wife have an argument about how often you leave your wet towel on the bathroom floor. You promise to do better, and you really begin to make an effort to hang up your towels. Then one morning, you are running late for work. You burst into the bathroom and there, lying on the floor for all the world to see, is *your wife's wet towel*. BUSTED!

Instantly your mind is enraged. Your thoughts start flying about how she is a hypocrite, how she's always getting on to you but she does the same things as you, how she doesn't notice how hard you're trying to change, how you're never picking up your wet towel ever again, and on and on.

Your body is geared up for battle, your blood pressure has rocketed, and you're making lists and stomping around the house.

But all your anger, indignation, and tough-guy talk is a complete waste of time.

A mindful approach would look something like this:

You see her wet towel on the floor, and as you begin to get insta-angry, you take a deep breath and hold it. You slowly let it out and drop your shoulders. You intentionally create space between what you feel and what you do or think next.

You hear the first thought about her being a hypocrite and you challenge it: *Is she really a hypocrite?* Not that you know of.

Then you ask yourself a second question: *I know a clean bathroom floor is important to her, so what in the world could have been going on for her to have forgotten her towel?*

Next, you redirect: *I'm going to reach out and remind her I love her and I'm here for her if she needs anything.* And then you pick up the towel and go about your day.

Your pulse rate barely changes. Your thoughts return to more important things like what's for lunch. You think of a hilarious joke.

See the difference?

The non-mindful approach is about fight or flight. The mindful approach is about prioritizing connection with your wife and creating a gap between the thoughts that pop into your mind and your body's response. When we practice this way of being, our brain actually grows new pathways to make this type of reaction easier and more automatic in the future.

Dr. Brewer says this about mindfulness:

> Meditation is like a gym for your brain, allowing you to build and strengthen your mindfulness muscles. Awareness also helps you pay attention to triggers and automatic reactions. . . . Mindfulness is about changing our relationship to those thoughts and emotions.[66]

In the context of anxiety, being mindful means listening to the alarms, asking why they're sounding, and looking for the root cause first.

Instead of running around trying to take out the batteries in the alarms, a mindful approach searches for the fire,

---

[66] Judson Brewer, *Unwinding Anxiety: Train Your Brain to Heal Your Mind* (New York: Avery, Penguin Random House, 2021), 86.

verifies whether the alarms are real, checks on anyone sleeping in the back of the burning house, and takes appropriate action depending on the answers.

RUN-IN WITH MY DAUGHTER *REIMAGINED*

According to Dr. Brewer, there are two key components to mindfulness—awareness and curiosity. He says this about awareness:

> If you aren't aware that you're doing something habitually, you will continue to do it habitually. . . . Building awareness through mindfulness helps you "pop the hood" on what's going on in your old brain. You can learn to recognize your habit loops while they're happening, rather than "waking up" at the end when you've almost crashed the car.[67]

Choosing to be mindful instead of reactive allows you to examine your body's response and your thoughts from a 30,000-foot view.

This perspective changes everything.

On that day my daughter lashed out, I allowed her to hurt my feelings. When she said she wished I never existed, *I chose to be bummed out. She didn't make me feel or do anything.*

My mind and body heard those words and were off to the races. My stomach dropped, my head got hot, and I

---

[67] Brewer, *Unwinding Anxiety*, 71–72.

immediately hid under a blanket of shame. My brain started making up stories: *You're a terrible father. Your little girl will grow up never wanting to know her dad. You have no business telling other people how to love or parent if that's how it is in your own home.*

But context was everything.

It was 5:15 in the morning.

I'd just returned from a multi-city speaking tour.

She was tired.

I was exhausted.

Oh, and she's FIVE!

There's a reason we don't let five-year-olds drive or buy beer. Because they're FIVE! Their brains aren't fully formed yet.

What if I stepped out on the porch, curious at the things a tired five-year-old says, and asked myself, *Do I really suck at being a dad?* The answer would have been a resounding no. I'm a pretty good dad.

And what if I'd taken that as a cue to consider how I could find time for us to connect, once we were both rested? I could lean into my role as her dad to make sure she felt loved, connected, and supported whether I was traveling or not. Thinking up strategies for deepening my connection with my daughter would have been a much more productive use of my time.

Or what if I'd chosen to skip my workout and instead grabbed breakfast for the family, and come back into the house a half-hour later with dance music blaring on my

Bluetooth speaker? What if I rearranged my lists and routines to include connection as the top priority?

This is choosing mindfulness.

MINDFULNESS IN REAL LIFE

Mindfulness is essential for choosing connection, choosing reality, choosing freedom. In fact, it's essential for all six
of our Daily Choices. But most of us live chained-up and
unfree lives, and we spend all available energy reacting to the
past or trying to anticipate the future. We don't know how—
we literally lack the skills—to be present where we are.

To be mindful, we must first become aware.

Awareness

Let's think about our lives in "react" mode:

Every dig from our annoying sibling or in-law is a personal attack on our ego. Every time someone tails us too
close in traffic, it's an affront. Every time somebody stares
past us when we're talking, leaves us off the invite list, or
gets frustrated with us because we didn't meet their deadlines, our bodies either start throwing punches or heading
underground before we even have a moment to think. We
impulse-buy, impulse-eat, impulse-email, impulse-retreat . . .
and then we do it again the next time. We are living unaware.

Anxiety is integrally linked to reactive living. Non-
anxious people aren't reactive. They are intentional. Anxious

and scared and unfree people, on the other hand, are ranting on social media or letting their middle finger fly at other drivers before even considering what happens next.

Reactivity can be big and loud. Anxious-reactivity can also be a quiet withdrawing from loved ones. Into isolation. A fading out. A sitting in the shadows. This is you when you disappear in a crowded room. Or you vanish while sitting at a table of people who love you deeply.

We sit at our desks and mindlessly fiddle with some work something-or-other instead of going to see our kids and hug our wives.

We bury ourselves in a book, or woodworking in the garage, or *Monday Night Football.*

We apply for job after job after job or look online for house after house instead of making the most of the homes and jobs we already have.

As Dr. Gabor Maté eloquently states, "Once I notice my programmed, defensive impulse to withdraw from intimacy and understand its source, I have some choice whether or not to act it out."[68]

Becoming aware is about recognizing your impulses and pausing to consider your next move. It's about being thoughtful, patient, and intentional about what you choose to say, think, or do next. This is the practice of stretching the gap between stimulus and response.

---

[68] Gabor Maté, *In the Realm of Hungry Ghosts: Close Encounters with Addiction* (Berkeley, CA: North Atlantic Books, 2010), 371.

Make no mistake, mindful awareness is scary and difficult.

Remember back to chapter 4: Choose Reality. It's scary to realize you're pulling away from your wife. Or you're unsure how to talk to your middle-school daughter. Or your heart-rate heads north of 100 beats per minute when you pull into the parking lot of your job site on Monday mornings. Or every time your dad calls, you automatically silence the phone and then feel a deep sense of shame.

Awareness can be terrifying. But it's one entry point for mindfully silencing the alarms.

Here's an example of awareness applied:

In a moment of intimate connection, your husband reaches over to grab your hand. For some reason, you think of the time he lied to you about his affair several years ago. It's like a lightning bolt to your mind. You catch your body pulling away from his touch. Even though you chose to stay and your marriage is better than it's been in years, pulling away is still your automated response. Your mind still starts telling stories.

But this time you choose something different.

This time, you're going to be mindful.

He reaches over to grab your hand, and while you instantly feel the familiar need to pull away, you catch your breath, hold it for a beat, and softly release it. You intentionally drop your shoulders. You loosen your jaw.

You don't rush a reaction. Instead, you gently ask yourself, "I wonder why my body is reacting as though I don't want to hold my husband's hand? I love him, and I know he loves me." And here's the magic question: *I wonder what my body is trying to protect me from right now?*

Maybe you are sensing, deep down inside, that your husband is acting like he did so many years ago when he was having an affair. Or maybe you've pulled away for so long that it doesn't even register anymore.

All of this begins with awareness.

Awareness of how your body is reacting to the stories your thoughts are concocting, and how your mind and your body are working (or not working) together. Awareness of the abuse, neglect, and injustice you're experiencing.

Everything begins with awareness.

This is a part of choosing mindfulness.

Curiosity

A second entry point into mindfulness as a way of life is curiosity.

Have you ever stopped for a moment to listen to the voice in your head? Ethan Kross, professor and best-selling author of *Chatter*, says, "A main culprit in keeping stress active is our negative verbal stream."[69]

Imagine yourself standing in line at your neighborhood grocery store. You're making faces back and forth with the little kid behind you when suddenly you hear a guy in front

---

[69] Ethan Kross, *Chatter: The Voice in Our Head, Why It Matters, and How to Harness It* (New York: Crown, 2022), 39.

of you screaming at the clerk. The clerk is a 60-year-old woman, moving slow and deliberate, clearly tired, but doing her best to greet each customer with a smile and a little bit of sunshine.

The customer is belligerent. He calls her stupid, slow, and worthless—and lets her know she has no business working when she clearly can't do the job right.

If you're like most decent people in the world, you would get involved. Some of you might step in and just deck the guy, sending him to the floor to look for his teeth. I'm not advising this plan, but I'd understand it. Others of you would signal for the manager, step in between the angry customer and the store clerk, or call security.

My point here is, almost everyone reading this would do something. Something big or something small . . . but something to stop the chaos.

Yet if you're like me, you talk *to yourself* like this ALL THE TIME!

The voice in your head never lets up. It's always telling you:

You're weird.

You're too fat.

You're never going to get out of this job . . . this town . . . this abusive marriage.

Only losers get divorced.

You don't have a shred of common sense.

Nobody would ever want you.

You're a bad mom.

And on and on.

Sometimes, in an effort to pump you up just enough for you to face the world, your inner voice blasts everyone around you. *They're* too fat, too weird; *they're* the losers. That inner voice is ruthless and unforgiving. It's always firing away, either at you or other people.

But that voice of judgment is paralyzing *you*.

This is the voice of your critical older brother. Your ex-boyfriend. This is the voice of your power-hungry pastor or your mean-girl friends, or your best friend who still struggles with addiction. This is the voice of your controlling boss or your never-happy in-laws. And over time, these voices—these stories you were told and born into and have lived—become the stories you tell yourself.

You start to hear them in your own voice. And they rattle about in your mind unchallenged.

Sometimes these voices aren't voices at all. They're intense feelings. They're emotional outbreaks. They're bodily responses: a tight chest, a crick in your neck, lower back pain, and more.

It's the erupting feeling that you need to get out of here.

That you need to run.

That no one can be trusted.

Once we become aware of the constant chattering, our next immediate challenge is to not instantly believe the voices.

This is the turn from judgment to curiosity.

Switching to a posture of curiosity instead of judging and complaining and criticizing could save your marriage, your relationship with your kids, your friendships, and the morale and camaraderie at work. When I think about cardiovascular disease, cancers, stroke, and blood pressure-related issues, choosing to see the world through a lens of curiosity might just save your life.

In his book *Unwinding Anxiety*, Dr. Brewer suggests an exercise for practicing curiosity. First, he recommends you find a peaceful, relaxing space where you can concentrate without distraction.[70] He then suggests recalling a time when you felt anxious and were compelled to act. Let's say you demolished half-a-dozen doughnuts. Or you lashed out at someone. Or you wept from deep inside your guts.

Whatever it is you're remembering, dial in on what you did—the actual actions you took following the triggering moment. Dr. Brewer recommends seeing if you can "relive that experience, focusing on what you felt right at the time when you were about to act out the habitual behavior. What did that urge to go ahead and 'do it' feel like?"[71] He goes on to suggest you find out where the urge shows up in your body: hunger in the stomach, your cheeks getting hot, your shoulders tightening up.

The goal here is to create space. Unchain yourself from automated responses, ask questions of yourself, and make

---

[70] All the moms with young kids just laughed and said, "Well, I'm out!" I know a distraction-free place feels like a faraway land filled with unicorns and flying fairies that fart gumdrops, but stay with me. It's worth figuring this part out.

[71] Brewer, *Unwinding Anxiety*, 183.

intentional choices about what you think and do next. Dr. Brewer remarks, "If you noticed that by being curious you just gained even a microsecond of being able to be with your thoughts, emotions, and body sensations more than you have in the past, you've just taken a huge leap forward."[72]

Additionally, here's an old cognitive behavioral technique I've used to free myself from my inner critic. I've also taught this to thousands of folks, including my own kids.

I want you to keep your notes app open on your phone. Or if you're a Luddite like me, carry a small notebook, journal, or notecard. When you have these moments of judgment, write down exactly what the inner voice is saying.

Here are some examples:

You really don't need a second cheeseburger.

I will never be a vice president.

My church would reject me if they knew everything about me.

Mom will die if we don't do Christmas at her house.

My husband is always going to be an embarrassment to me because he won't ever lose the weight.

The world as we know it will be gone 10 years from now.

My wife left the gas tank on empty because she's lazy and trying to make me late.

I'm going to be in debt for the rest of my life.

Write down these thoughts. The judgments, the complaints, the grenades. Literally get them out of your body and onto the paper. Then pause, take a moment, and read them.

---

[72] Brewer, 185.

As you read them, **demand evidence**. Are the things circulating throughout your mind and body true? Can you confirm the accuracy of the poison pulsing through your veins?

Sometimes the answer will be yes. I can't think of a time when I *need* a second cheeseburger. I need to turn away from the drive-thru. But the vast majority of the time, demanding evidence from these thoughts and actions serves as the great diffuser. It literally takes the air out of the habit loop and stops urges dead in their tracks.

Being curious helps you arrive at truth and a calmer response much faster than a mindless rush to judgment.

- Is the guy who just cut you off in traffic really a drugged-out scumbag who has no regard for human life? Or is he trying to get to the hospital as quickly as he can before his wife passes away?
- Did your husband leave dishes in the sink because he's selfish and doesn't care about you, or have you never told him that putting the dishes away makes you feel seen and loved, especially when you're exhausted?
- Is your co-worker who disagrees with you about how Jesus would respond to a social issue a stupid, woke idiot or a callous, conservative moron? Or have they educated themselves on the topic and simply come to a different conclusion than you?

Or, as I asked myself, *John, are you really a terrible father? Or have you just been on the road for a few days, and your five-year-old daughter legitimately misses you and doesn't have the words to say, "Daddy, my heart, mind, and spirit don't feel right when you're not here"?*

You have to examine your thoughts like you might examine your spending. You have to challenge them to see what's real or whether your mind is just making up stories.

Sometimes you'll realize you're being a jerk. That you jumped the gun, or weren't being completely honest, or did something you shouldn't have done. What often follows awareness and curiosity is a spirit of humility. A spirit of forgiveness or repentance. Empathy and compassion.

This is acting like an adult, in a world populated by people acting like grown-up children.

After curiosity comes a recognition of common humanity and vulnerability. It becomes an opportunity to learn, to challenge, and to find places to connect.

A spirit of curiosity is an important touchstone on the path of the non-anxious life.

Don't ever forget: Awareness and curiosity can save your life.

A FEW REMINDERS ABOUT MINDFULNESS

Mindfulness is a way of being. It's an orientation toward the world, your thoughts, and your reactions. It's also a thing you do. Dr. Brewer reports, "There are now hundreds of published scientific papers on the clinical efficacy and even the neuroscience behind mindfulness."[73] We know it works, but not like turning a wrench, popping a pill, or having surgery.

Mindfulness lifts your eyes away from yourself so you can take in the world around you. It helps you shift from reacting to responding. For you Type A's out there, or for you hard-charging CEOs, mindfulness is not a competition. It's not something you try to win.

Mindfulness is also not some gooey way to relax and avoid feeling. It's not about trying to circumvent pain or leave your human form to imagine yourself sitting criss-cross-applesauce on a cloud. Mindfulness can be as much about putting your foot down and starting over as it is about learning and listening.

Mindfulness and Feelings

Challenging your thoughts—taking the time to lengthen the gap between something happening and your response—is brave and difficult. It's very, very hard. So don't be lulled into thinking mindfulness is easy or passive. It's real work!

Being curious about your body's responses can birth some truly scary truths. Maybe you *aren't* safe. Maybe he *is* trying to hurt and demean you. Maybe you *are* being irresponsible.

And sometimes those truths call for intentional actions in return. Sometimes our impulse to back out or run is right.

---

[73] Brewer, *Unwinding Anxiety*, 241.

Occasionally, we may need to plant a flag and declare our intent to die on this hill.

Our feelings can be loud and they don't always tell the truth.

But sometimes they do.

I believe, with all of my being, we should listen to our gut. We shouldn't trust it without question, but we should certainly listen to it. Always.

Our thoughts trigger feelings, and feelings are simply traffic signals telling us to slow down, go, or come to a complete stop. Best-selling author Melody Beattie writes,

> Our feelings are very important. They count. They matter. . . . Repressing or denying feelings can lead to headaches, stomach disorders, backaches . . . [and] into trouble with overeating, undereating, alcohol and other drug use, compulsive sexual behaviors, compulsive spending, not sleeping enough, sleeping too much, obsessing, controlling gestures, and other compulsive behaviors. . . . But, feelings are not the end all and be all to living. Feelings must not dictate or control our behaviors, but we can't ignore [them].[74]

The goal is to be aware of our body's responses, our thoughts, and our feelings. To notice them, and not simply be

---

[74] Melody Beattie, *Codependent No More: How to Stop Controlling Others and Start Caring for Yourself* (Center City, MN: Hazelden Publishing, 1992), 143–45.

in a constant state of reaction. And when we do notice them, not to immediately accept them as the truth of all truths, or judge them—or ourselves—as stupid, lame, or crazy. This is the importance of curiosity over judgment.

Mindfulness and Meditation

I highly recommend some form of meditation as a way of practicing being mindful. I've been practicing meditation, contemplative introspection, prayer, and other ancient ways of "sacred knowing" for many years. This has changed my life. Personally, I credit mindfulness, meditation, and prayer with helping heal my mind and turning the anxiety alarms way, way down.

I usually use an app on my phone and some headphones, and I create a little space in my basement. Some days I feel like I'm meditating deeply, and other days I feel like I'm wasting my time. But as I said above, it's not a competition. It's a practice. When I was super-anxious, I tried to make meditation solve everything. I tried to use it as a balm or a medicine. Meditation doesn't work like that.

Meditation is like spending time with an old friend. After several cups of coffee and several hours of engaging conversation, you stand up to find you are more at peace than before you sat down.

Dr. Gabor Maté has said, "I realized that my expectations for meditation practice had been too harsh—on myself. I wanted to be good at it, I wanted spiritually uplifting things to happen, I wanted deep insights to arise. I know now it's a gentle process."[75]

Meditation is gentle.

Prayer is surrendering.

Mindfulness is a slower, less aggressive approach.

This is the path to the non-anxious life.

CHOOSE MINDFULNESS

Chapter Summary and Next Steps

Summary:

- Mindfulness is the practice of consciously stretching the gap between stimulus (i.e., the thing that makes you mad) and your response (punching a hole in the wall or walking away).
- Being mindful of your thoughts is about owning each thought as it enters your mind and being intentional about how, or if, you choose to respond.
- Two keys to being mindful are awareness and curiosity.
- Awareness is the intentional feeling of the positive and negative things in your life and your body's automated responses.
- Mindful curiosity is the choice to seek understanding, calm, and inquiry over judgment, reaction, and response.

---

[75] Maté, *In the Realm of Hungry Ghosts*, 372.

Things to Do:

- Go to johndelony.com/resources for a free guided meditation to help you lean in, listen, and clear your head.
- Keep a thoughts journal. When a negative or troubling thought zaps into your head, stop and write it down.
- Commit to being mindful of thoughts and actions that contribute to you being less joyful, kind, and patient. Consider negative media consumption, toxic relationships, and your own whining and complaining.
- Commit to ending negative self-talk and speaking negatively about others.
- Never keep secrets. Secrets get bound up in the body and become automated responses.
- Practice pausing before reacting . . . about anything. Create response rules for yourself. For instance: You will take 24 hours before responding to a hurtful email. You will only respond to text messages twice a day. If someone says something negative about you, you will take one hour before responding.
- Make a list of your needs, your desires, and who you can share them with.

Ask Yourself:

- What are 5–10 things that make me angry or upset?
  - How do I instantly respond to each of these occurrences?

- When do my responses resolve the situation and make me feel peaceful and calm? When do my responses make a situation worse and make me feel activated and upset over the long-term?
- What are a few feelings I've been experiencing regularly over the past few weeks/months/years? Where are these feelings coming from?
  - In direct words, what stories arise in me regarding those feelings (examples: *I'm a terrible mom. My wife hates me. I'll never be able to please my mother-in-law*, etc.).
  - Demand evidence from the stories. Go through each story one by one, and ask: Is this story true? Then explore the evidence about whether it is accurate.

Additional Resources:

- Go to johndelony.com/resources for a list of books, podcasts, and tools to help you start down the path toward a non-anxious life.

THE
6 DAILY CHOICES

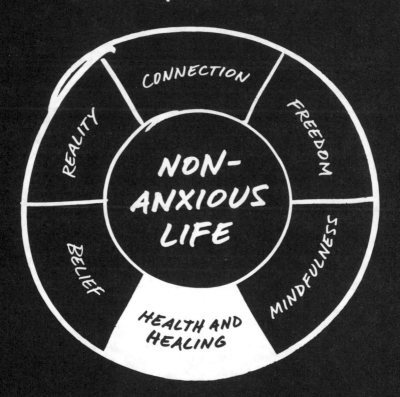

CHAPTER 8

CHOOSE HEALTH AND HEALING

About 10 years ago, as I've shared, I was buried with anxiety. I couldn't sleep. I'd isolated myself and become radioactive emotionally. Once I started discovering that the problem was within me—and not everyone else—I decided to take matters into my own hands. I was going to solve my issues with my intellect.

I resolved to think my way out of anxiety.

I was privileged to work at a university. This meant I had access to research journals, books, and experts of all kinds, from all over the world. Besides talking (and talking) with every educated person I could connect with, I started reading everything I could get my hands on and listening to as many seminars and lectures as I could download. I studied nutrition, science, mental health, and cardiovascular health.

I was obsessed with my subject matter. I wanted to know how the HPA axis worked, I wanted to learn all about the sympathetic and parasympathetic nervous system, the amygdala, and on and on. I was determined to know whatever there was to know about anxiety.[76]

I didn't realize it at the time, but I was swimming in the Enlightenment reductionism that has haunted science and philosophy for centuries. Here's the idea of Enlightenment reductionism: You can best know about something by taking it apart, down to its smallest pieces, and studying those individual parts. Truth is found in the pieces, not in how they all work together.

In this way of learning, water isn't the life-force of all living things and also a powerful destructive force; it is two parts hydrogen and one part oxygen. Thoughts and dreams are neuronal conversations across synapses. Anger and fear are part cortisol, part norepinephrine, plus a dose of *blah, blah, blah.* The brilliant poet and author Rebecca Reynolds cursed scientists for turning our romantic thoughts of stars into seeing them as they are—just balls of burning gas.[77]

I thought if I took apart anxiety and knew how it worked in my body—how it activated hormones, neurotransmitters,

---

[76] I'm sure this goes without saying, but I was a bundle of joy to be around during this time. Just a ray of freakin' sunshine, reflecting into a giant dumpster fire.

[77] Gone are the days of "Twinkle, twinkle little star / How I wonder what you are." Now I know. And it's not super-romantic. I've got to agree with Rebecca. *Damn scientists.*

and neuromodulators—I could finally understand, and fix, my broken brain.

Likewise, when it came to "fixing my mental health" (which is a statement I hate with all my heart because it is not medically, spiritually, or mechanistically correct). I assumed if I could just get my thoughts in the right order, I would be all better. I thought getting well was equal parts brain chemistry and correctly aligning the right thoughts to do the right things.

Turns out that's kinda-sorta true.

But I completely missed the point.

I bought the lie that I could outthink my anxiety. I really believed I could spin-move my way around my physical and mental life in order to shut off the alarms.

And all the while, I basically quit exercising. I was eating junk, both in quality and quantity. As I mentioned in chapter 6, I was perpetually racing around and late to everything, borrowing money, and living with no margin in just about every way.

It was like the smoke alarms were going off in my kitchen, and I decided to Google "fire" and start reading. Sure, I learned a lot about fire, but my house still burned down around me.

In order to create a non-anxious life, and in order to give your body a chance to function as it should—as an integrated, well, and whole system—you must *Choose Health and Healing*.

You have to take care of your body and recover from past traumas.

You have to step into new relationships and grieve old ones.

You have to incorporate exercise and movement into each day.

You may need a therapist.

You certainly need some blood work.

You have to choose to believe you're worth being well.

This path is painful. And wildly uncomfortable. Choosing health and healing is often two steps forward, six steps back. You realize you're carrying trauma, and your life has been reduced to heavy feelings and a hurting back and knees. You're not caring for your one precious body. You've stopped changing the oil, and you have two flat tires, and you're wondering why the car isn't driving well.

Trauma and past emotional hurts sound the anxiety alarms. Physical pain, poor nutrition, poor health, or the things we do to artificially energize or dampen ourselves may also trigger the anxiety alarms. Because we are not safe.

If you want to build a non-anxious life, part of your journey must include healing from trauma, a focus on your physical and mental health, and finding safety.

CHOOSING HEALING

Most of us show up to our everyday lives carrying old traumas, generational family stories and experiences, and pre-programmed physical responses stored in our bodies. For many of us, our body's responses to these stories kept us alive.

But as we've grown up, our bodies are responding to per-ceived threats that may no longer be present.

Trauma is our body's response in the present to things that happened in our past. Those experiences begin to cause problems in our personal, professional, and family relationships.

As we've seen thus far, creating a non-anxious life is a tough row to hoe. And creating a non-anxious life while daily trying to live with past trauma is near-impossible.

Listen, countless things have happened to you that you did not want, desire, or ask for.

You did not choose to be sexually assaulted.

You did not choose for your dad to leave you when you were seven.

You did not choose to see your friend shot down and killed while you were both on deployment.

You did not choose for the economy to implode, or to get the email confirming your layoff, or to have an ego-maniacal boss.

You did not choose for people to hate you or exclude you because of your skin color, your financial position, your culture, or who you love.

You did not choose your genetics, the traumas of your great-grandparents, or the hell your mom lived in while she was pregnant with you.

You did not choose so much that has happened to you in your life. Yet here you are. All the roads of your past, and of your family's past, have led to this moment.

To this place.

Trauma

Many of us hear the word *trauma* and we think of the big, scary experiences. In the nerd world, we call the nuclear-blast type of experiences *acute trauma*. Acute trauma is the big car crash, the sexual molestation, the death of your husband, or your mom's stomachache that turned out to be stage IV cancer. As I mentioned earlier, our bodies put a GPS pin in these moments and devise defensive, evasive maneuvers in an attempt to never be hurt by these same things again.

But there are other types of trauma. *Secondary trauma* is when your body responds to the steady stream of pain you absorb through proximity to other hurting people. Like serving as a nurse or a teacher or a police officer and stepping into the gnarliest, rawest scenes imaginable. Think social workers, counselors, schoolteachers, and ministers too. Think lawyers, doctors, and dentists. All these folks enter into the pain of others for a living. Over time, this has an impact on their bodies as well.

Trauma can even be *neglect*—the things that should have happened to you but didn't.

As a child, you should have been fed, clothed, housed, and loved. You should have been told you had value. You should have been lovingly held and warmly touched, and your mother should have been closely attuned to your expressions, your body, and your needs. She should have stared into your eyes and told you how loved you are.

You should have been believed. Your father should have helped you, roughhoused with you, and every day said some version of "I love you, and every single day I thank God for picking me to be your dad."

Trauma can also be *collective* (think Holocaust survivors, war veterans, or car-wreck survivors)—or *cumulative* (think the little insults you endured for years on the bus and on the ballfield that added up to how much you loathe yourself as an adult today).

Trauma is not only your body's present response to things that happened in the past, but it's an overloading of your body's ability to respond. It's emergency mode, and it expresses itself in many different ways. Our hearts pound, we get that sinking feeling in our stomachs. We get sick. Our backs hurt. Our necks hurt. We cry, sometimes for seemingly no reason. We struggle with insomnia or our legs feel like lead when we're trying to get out of bed.

Do you see the connection? Our body's trauma responses sound the anxiety alarms.

In order to build a non-anxious life, you and I must be willing to heal old wounds and do the hard work in therapy to learn how to re-train our bodies as to what safety and connection feel like.

Maybe you always smelled alcohol on your dad's breath when he came home, kicking and screaming his way through the house. And maybe now, years later, your body flinches when your loving husband leans over to whisper in your ear how much he loves you and you catch a whiff of his glass of bourbon from earlier in the evening.

Your body can't smell that scent without screaming at you to RUN AWAY! And your husband experiences your response as a move away from him, not your abusive father.

Maybe as a kid, you were told you were stupid, or that your feelings were in the way and didn't count. You were told, "That doesn't hurt!" or "Quit making such a big deal about things that don't matter," or "I'M GONNA GIVE YOU SOMETHING TO CRY ABOUT!" And maybe now, your body has lost its ability to listen to itself, and to feel, and to honestly communicate feelings.

Your body cannot be vulnerable and speak your needs out loud because expression meant getting hit or being yelled at or shamed. And now the person you love most in the world is experiencing your non-responsiveness as rejection.

Or maybe you grew up in scarcity. You never missed a meal, but fights about money were constant and pervasive. There was almost-daily tension and pressure related to money. And now, 17 years later, even though you're making a decent salary and you're current on your mortgage payments, to even think of discussing compensation with your boss sends your pulse rate through the roof. The entire week before your job review, you're a wreck. Night sweats, a constant headache, nausea. Your body cannot talk about money without either gearing up for a fight or wanting to run and hide.

Deeply internalize this:

You are worth more than the worst thing that's ever happened to you.

You are worth more than the worst thing you've ever done.

You are worth more than the stories you inherited.

These things do not have to be your legacy or your identity. And . . .

You cannot change what happened to you.

That moment is gone.

You can only choose what happens next.

The Choices

Unless you're some kind of robotic superhuman, you can't simply snap your fingers and Control-Alt-Delete the years of layers your body has built up to protect you.

In the beginning, we can't choose how our body responds. But we can choose healing.

- We can choose to see a professional counselor.
- We can grieve the life we wanted but up until now haven't had.
- We can move out.
- We can say yes. Or no.
- We can begin to develop and practice boundaries.
- We can see a medical doctor and get our blood work done. Or meet with a psychiatrist and start a medication.

- We can hire a personal trainer, utilize free YouTube videos in our garage or bedroom, and stop mainlining doomsday information on 24/7 news channels.
- We can forgive.
- We can write that letter.
- We can take classes. Sign up for the training. Finish the degree.
- We can make a move, start a new job.

Choosing healing is about deciding to face your anxiety and trauma. This is about changing your family tree. Creating a new legacy. As the best-selling author and master therapist Terrence Real says, "Family dysfunction rolls down from generation to generation, like a fire in the woods, taking down everything in its path until one person in one generation has the courage to turn and face the flames. That person brings peace to their ancestors and spares the children that follow."[78]

If you're the first person in your family to choose healing, you'll have scars. You'll have pain and scrapes and burns as you battle the forest fire and carve a new path in the wilderness.

But your children won't.

And their kids and neighbors, and people you've never met, will walk on the new paths you've illuminated in the darkness.

---

[78] Check out the home page of Terrence Real, https://terryreal.com /trauma/.

Choosing healing is about doing what it takes to feel at home in your body.

To feel valued and truly loved in your relationships.

To feel your unique purpose and be firmly anchored to your values.

This is the path you must walk for a non-anxious life.

CHOOSING HEALTH

When I talk about health, I am referring to your physical body. I know mental and physical and relational and spiritual and emotional health are intertwined. But for this one section, I am going to focus exclusively on your physical health.

In order to have anxiety alarms that work properly, that ring when they should, and that last over time, you have to maintain the system. You must make sure your home is secure and strong, the wiring is good, the batteries are fresh, and the alarm system receives maintenance. You must choose to take care of your body.

A cornerstone of the non-anxious life is the daily choice to honor, love, and maintain your physical health. How you move. How you are able to get up off the floor, lift heavy objects, or get up and down a flight of stairs. How you make love, dance, run, or are able to catch yourself from falling. What you eat and how you nourish your body. How many cups of coffee and energy drinks you consume. How you touch and are touched. It's about sleep and rest and intentionally setting aside time for your body to recover, renew, and recharge. Your physical body is about your nervous system, your muscles and skeleton, cardiovascular disease, dementia, and cancer. In short, can you do the things you want to do, or do you have physical limitations?

There are countless studies correlating physical health and mental health. It is virtually impossible to be well and whole when you're in chronic physical pain. It is almost impossible to be well and whole when you're not able to play with your kids, when you're too tired to go dancing, or you're too out of shape to finish a round of golf. It's hard to laugh from your guts when you can't breathe. Being unable to do what you want to do makes living a well and non-anxious life extremely difficult. Not impossible, but very challenging.

Before I move on to action steps, I want to acknowledge my most enduring friend on the planet. Ryan was in a devastating car accident the week after he graduated from college. He suffered a traumatic brain injury and has had severe mobility impairment for decades. He can't go anywhere without his wheelchair and someone to help him out.

He still goes to physical therapy on a regular basis. He works harder than any gym-rat I know. Am I suggesting that he is going to have a much more difficult time building a non-anxious life than I am?

Yes.

His road has been infinitely more difficult than mine. But every single day he can be found with his amazing brother, his caretaker, his mom and stepdad, and multiple professionals working to help him slowly regain some function across parts of his body. His reality is that his journey is more difficult than mine. But he still has to get in the saddle and give it a go.

He inspires me, a fully able-bodied man, to not waste my ability to run and jump and dance. Why in the world would I sit around and play video games when I have been blessed with the opportunity to be fully active and seek adventures?

How to Choose Health

Our physical bodies are a mess. A quick glance at the actuarial tables regarding obesity, cardiovascular disease, diabetes, Alzheimer's and dementia, cancer, and other modern diseases is enough to send most of us running for the hills. The environment we've created for our bodies is contributing to our deteriorating health.

Michael Easter, professor and best-selling author of *The Comfort Crisis* writes,

The second great change in human fitness began around 1850. It marked the start of the Industrial Revolution, and today, just 13.7 percent of jobs require the same heavy work as our past days of farming. Roughly three-quarters of jobs are now sedentary, and we're sitting more every year. Over the last decade, the average American added another hour of daily sitting. Adults now sit for six and a half hours, while kids sit more than eight (the removal of recess hasn't helped, either).[79]

For the sake of simplicity, let's divide up our health into a few buckets: movement and exercise, sleep, nutrition, and professional support.

Almost overnight, we've stopped moving. We don't exercise—or when we do, as Easter points out, we do it in air-conditioned gyms, in specialized group classes, on smooth surfaces, in crafted, padded shoes. So while the exercise is a good thing, we're not getting as much benefit from our movement as we used to.

We also don't sleep. We have come to view sleep as a luxury or a reward, not the necessity it is. And if you're a single mom working three jobs to try to pay what has become an outrageous rent, sleep is but a dream. If you're the CEO of a Fortune 500 company, it sounds heroic to proclaim, "You'll sleep when you're dead!" But our lack of sleep is destroying our health and frazzling our bodies and minds.

In fact, it's killing us.

And for those of us who understand the value and importance of exercise, navigating the ocean of misinformation is a nightmare. A quick glance through social media, YouTube, or a local bookstore yields conflicting claims about what workouts we should be doing, how often, in what ways, and so

---

[79] Michael Easter, *The Comfort Crisis: Embrace Discomfort to Reclaim Your Wild, Happy, Healthy Self* (New York: Rodale Books, 2021), 225.

on. So much bickering about cardio versus weight-lifting; carnivore versus vegan; supplementation and boosters; free weights versus Nautilus-type machines; running outside versus a treadmill versus an elliptical trainer. I've been lifting and exercising regularly for more than three decades, and even I get overwhelmed with all the nonsense. I sometimes want to just blow off my workout and inhale a bag of gummy candies.

Speaking of gummy candies, our understanding of nutritional science is an absolute dumpster fire. Few things have been more misunderstood, misrepresented, and flat-out lied about than nutrition science and the related nutrition industry.

If you're like me, you don't know what to eat, how much to eat, when to eat, and whether it should be organic, gluten-free, fat-free, sugar-free—or maybe all the above. Bottom line: Our bodies are not designed for a steady stream of readily available foods acquired with little to no effort. We consume way too many calories, through both eating and drinking. My good friend, Dr. Layne Norton (an international expert on exercise and nutrition) points out that we major in the minors. For example, we'll read up on whether to be vegan or Keto, or whether sugar-free has any merit; meanwhile, we're doing whatever we can to avoid the unsexy discipline of training consistently, exercising regularly, and being mindfully aware of our calorie intake.

This is one area where, in recent years, I have learned a great deal and have changed my mind in significant ways. Now, instead of engaging in the Diet Religion Wars, I track my macros, eat when I'm hungry, and keep an eye on my caloric intake. And I am very graceful with myself when I choose to succumb to the occasional gummy bear/marshmallow bender.

If you'll allow me to oversimplify millions of pages of scientific literature and thousands of years of common sense, here are the key takeaways for choosing health:

Exercise

Dr. Peter Attia, a world-renowned physician, longevity expert, and best-selling author, often describes exercise as the single-most important longevity drug in the world. He explains that there isn't a drug known to man that decreases all-cause mortality (the likelihood that you'll die) better than exercise. This is especially true for those who go from little-to-no-movement to being somewhat fit. You must regularly and consistently exercise and move your body. Period.

I could cite countless studies on the massive mental- and physical-health benefits of all types of exercise, from movement-based practices like yoga and dance to weight-lifting, cardio, high-intensity training, and low-level walking. Dr. Wendy Suzuki and Dr. Thomas Joiner each report in their own respective work that exercise—even movement as simple as walking—can strengthen the part of the brain responsible for threat assessment and evaluation.

In discussing the important role movement and exercise play in reducing or eliminating anxiety, Dr. Suzuki notes, "It is very powerful to get sensitized to the mood boost and anxiety-busting effects of movement."[80] Exercise changes the brain in remarkable ways, helping with attention, depression, and of course, anxiety. In addition to Dr. Attia, I have found trustworthy information on the topic of exercise from experts such as Dr. Norton, Dr. Andy Galpin, Dr. Huberman, as well as information from the Mind Pump Media team.[81]

The takeaway: *Do some sort of movement or exercise every single day.*

Sleep

Dr. Matthew Walker, best-selling author, professor, and world-renowned sleep researcher would say sleep is a close, close second on the list of the most important wellness and longevity interventions. Loss of sleep, poor sleep, and insomnia are directly linked to anxiety and anxiety-related disorders. It's fair to say that the less sleep you get, the more anxious you're bound to feel.[82]

---

[80] Wendy Suzuki, *Good Anxiety: Harnessing the Power of the Most Misunderstood Emotion* (New York: Atria Books, 2021), 222.

[81] Check out Mind Pump Media team's radio show/podcast dedicated to providing truthful information about health and fitness—as well as a lot of entertainment. I love these guys and what they teach.

[82] Dr. Matthew Walker has authored numerous articles and created a bunch of videos on the science of sleep. I don't have the words to

I cannot stress this point enough: Very few of us get enough sleep. If you think you're doing great on four or five or even six hours of sleep, you're lying to yourself. If you have even a single drink close to bedtime, take hypnotic sleep medications, or stay up until midnight interacting with some sort of screen, your sleep will be dysregulated and disrupted. Do this over a short period of time and you're choosing to be irritable, forgetful, erratic, anxious, and feel off your game. Do this over the long-term and you're choosing to die early. The reams of scientific data back me up.

The takeaway: *Seek to get 7-9 hours of sleep every single night.* Build your life around adequate sleep. Make it a top, top, top priority. (Unless of course you have toddlers in the house. In that case, may the Force be with you.)

Nutrition

When it comes to nutrition, I know enough to say very little here.

Broadly speaking, you can't go wrong eating real, unprocessed (whole) foods. But you also won't suddenly die if you consume appropriate amounts of processed foods. Eat enough protein to fuel your body, and get enough carbohydrates and fats (I know those two words trigger different people in different ways). If you're an athlete, work closely

---

communicate how important this research and information (and just plain sleep!) is when it comes to your well-being.

with a coach or trainer to dial in your caloric needs with your specific training and performance goals. If you're a regular person like me, seek to get the right number of macros (protein, carbohydrates, fats) within the right number of calories for your body. Again, experts like Dr. Attia, Dr. Norton, Dr. Huberman, and others have been key resources for me.

One thing I can share is that sometimes feeling anxious is more about two energy drinks and five cups of coffee than it is about anything else. Caffeine and other stimulants can easily ramp up our bodies and mimic the feelings of anxiety. As you look into your own health and healing, consider a 30-day fast from caffeine. If you're like me, this is akin to torture, especially for the first two weeks or so. But it's worth discovering, via elimination followed by slow reintroduction, whether your body is sensitive to stimulants.

Professional Support

And finally, it's important to seek the advice of medical professionals on some sort of regular basis. Get regular blood work done. If you want to go deeper, add genetic testing and other medical tests. Go to the dentist. Get your moles and skin checked. Schedule a colonoscopy as early as your doctor will allow. Learn your family history. Take ownership of your health, and partner with trained professionals who went to med school or dental school and who spend more time with patients than on their social media channel.

For you and me who are just trying to design and build a non-anxious life, we need to know this: Caring for our one precious body with daily movement, great sleep, a good diet, and knowing professionals is critical.

Caring for ourselves is a choice.

SEEKING SAFETY

Underneath the charge to focus on health and healing is the single, unifying cornerstone of the non-anxious life: safety.

Ultimately, all of what we're doing here is creating an ecosystem or environment for our bodies that is safe. An environment that is anchored. Reliable. Stable. Connected.

What does this mean in the real world?

You may have to finally leave for good when he hits you.

You may have to tell her that her reckless spending terrifies you.

You may have to never do birthdays with your dad again until he agrees to stop going ballistic when he doesn't get his way.

You may have to quit your job because your body is telling you it can no longer handle the toll of the work, the overbearing boss, or the cutthroat industry.

You may have to take a leave of absence and go to rehab.

You may have to move out for 30 days until she agrees to get sober.

You are worth being safe. You must love yourself and your kids enough to be safe.

Beyond all the topics I discuss in this book, know that your safety and well-being are paramount. They're everything. If you're ever feeling anxious and you don't know where to start, ask yourself, "Am I safe right now?"

Answer this question honestly and it will give you direction. Either toward something or away from something. This question will light your path, even in the darkest times.

FINAL THOUGHTS

Before we leave this chapter, there are a few important ideas I want to pass along.

First, there's a difference between choosing to be healed—past tense—and choosing healing as a life direction in the present and into the future.

Unfortunately, you can't just snap your fingers and be healed. I would go as far as to suggest that we're never really "healed" in the past tense, as if our bodies never again call on old stories, old attachment issues, or old insecurities. We will constantly be faced with new challenges, responses to old traumas, and the struggles of life in today's world. And our brain and body will always be seeking to protect us, in whatever ways they know how.

So, let's shift out of one-and-done thinking.

You will never have one workout that is so successful, you can take the next month off from exercise.

You will never consume such a healthy meal that you can

mainline caramel-covered marshmallows for the following two weeks and not pay a price.

You'll never be so completely through with your past that you won't occasionally, randomly, find yourself sad or crying. Or suddenly click into exhaustion or a headache or anger.

Sometimes staying up way too late is necessary. Or completely worth the price you'll pay for the next few days. And sometimes, you'll just pop up awake for the night after only sleeping for a couple hours.

This is life.

And so perfection isn't the goal here.

Consistency is.

Bravery is.

Discipline is.

Co-creating a plan with experts and friends and family members and then sticking to it is.

This is about long-term life change. You will continue to take actions, challenge your thoughts, and seek healing and health every single day. For the rest of your life.

I know it sounds daunting. I'm living this with you. I know.

But I promise it's worth it.

I promise you're worth it.

And I promise you and your body can handle it. Especially if you just keep taking the next step in front of you. Just keep moving forward.

Second, I have left a lot on the cutting room floor here. There is so much more to the health and healing story. For further reading, I want to point you in the direction of my first book, *Own Your Past, Change Your Future*, which is a long-form discussion about trauma, the stories you were told, the stories you were born into, and how to heal from your past to create an entirely new future. Additionally, I've included a number of books that taught, inspired, and transformed my thinking and actions around healing from trauma, mental-health challenges, and overall life change. Check out some of the books and authors on that list. My hope is they will help you change your life like they helped me change mine.

ALMOST THERE!

So now we have one more choice to make.

You are working to create a non-anxious life. You're establishing an environment where your alarm systems aren't always trying to get your attention. You are choosing freedom, you're owning reality, you have friends and support networks, you're becoming mindful of your thoughts and your body's responses. You've also decided to prioritize health, healing, and safety. You're almost there.

To truly create and live a non-anxious life, we will have to turn and stare down the most enticing, addictive, and powerful cultural blowtorch that is burning so many of us from the inside out.

It's up next, in chapter 9.

─────── **CHOOSE HEALTH AND HEALING** ───────

Chapter Summary and Next Steps

Summary:

- Your physical health may be contributing to feelings of anxiety and chronic stress. Certain physical conditions can activate your body's anxiety alarms.
- Your mental and emotional health plays a key role in feelings of anxiety and overstimulation.
- If you have historical trauma or you're working through mental illness, your body will continue to sound the alarms of safety and disconnection.
- Healing from past traumas, physical pain, and relational pain takes time. Often, a lifetime.

Things to Do:

- Do some sort of movement or exercise every single day. We've created a 30-day activity tracker available at johndelony.com/resources to help log your progress.
- Get 7–9 hours of sleep each night.
- Consider drastically reducing your alcohol intake.
- Go see a doctor and have appropriate blood work done.
- Make an appointment with your dentist.
- If you have trauma, relationship challenges, or other emotional-health challenges, go see a counselor.
- Commit to doing whatever it takes to get well. Even if it means putting yourself in a safe position to leave

your job, go to rehab, or enter an in-patient treatment facility. Make getting well a top priority.

Ask Yourself:

- Am I incorporating exercise or movement into every single day?
- How is my emotional health? How is my relational health?
- Do I have the resources in place (doctor, dentist, counselor, minister) to get well?
- Do I have financial resources, insurance, or other local support for the care I need? How can I secure these additional resources?
- Am I committed to getting well, even if it means removing unsafe, abusive, or toxic people, behaviors, or environments from my life? Do I love myself enough to do whatever it takes to be well? Why or why not?

Additional Resources:

- Go to johndelony.com/resources for a list of books, podcasts, and tools to help you start down the path toward a non-anxious life.

THE 6 DAILY CHOICES

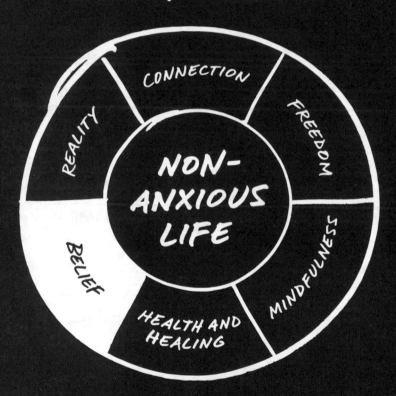

CHAPTER 9

CHOOSE BELIEF

Once a year, my colleagues and I head to our friend and boss's lake house for a time of retreat, planning, and hanging out. This year, before we got together, the leader of our team sent out an email inviting us to participate in an activity centered around my most paralyzing fear.

Before I tell you my fear, you need to understand this: I used to dive into swamps and ditches to catch snakes—I sold them to a pet store as a part-time job in high school. I've had adventures with alligators in the wild, caught sharks while wade-fishing, and trained with SWAT teams and professional MMA fighters. Professionally, I have intervened in domestic disputes, been in live-shooter situations, and spoken to audiences in the thousands and radio audiences in the millions. I've even talked to both of my kids about sex.

Here's my point: I'm not scared of much. Very little, in fact. But I am terrified, deep in my bones, of heights.

I don't like climbing on ladders, changing light bulbs, or being over six feet tall. I try not to even look over the second-story railing at my friend's house. I don't climb on roofs, and I sure don't like sitting in a tree stand during bow season.

I. Hate. Heights.

And then our team leader invited us to go skydiving.

Even reading his email invite gave me sweats. Skydiving is profound madness. Insanity. I would never do it.

I remember sitting at my desk at home, heart racing, and tentatively typing two words:

I'm in.

I was torn between two of my core values: Always run into your fears, not away from them; and DO NOT DIE FROM FALLING.

I chose to face my fears.

I didn't sleep well in the days leading up to the jump. I actively prayed for tornadoes, torrential rains, or a pre-jump plane malfunction. On the day of the dive, I had one thought the whole time I was getting geared up, putting my goggles on, and tightening my straps: *What are you doing? WHAT ARE YOU DOING?*

We all boarded the old, slow, metal tanker plane. It was sealed with duct tape on the inside.[83] Seriously. We meandered up to 14,000 feet, and the muscled-up former elite military officer who was leading my tandem jump casually

---

[83] Not hyperbole. I hate it when people say "literally," but the plane *literally* had parts on the inside held together by duct tape.

clicked us tightly together. He was chill. I was not. I was grateful to be anchored to him.

When it was our turn, we awkwardly hobble-walked over to the open airplane cargo door and held for a count.

And then,

We jumped.

I fell. Fast.

After quickly reaching terminal velocity, the world and the wind and the universe seemed to level out. Everything slowed down. It was one of the most transcendent, spiritual moments of my life. I will never forget staring over the horizon, realizing just how miniscule and unimportant I was. How dependent I was on someone else's care and concern. How free I was. Anchored into the professionals who stuffed the parachute, and the masterful veteran who was guiding me down, I simply let go into a reality bigger than my fears and my attempt to control them all.

This surrender of imaginary control is belief.

Belief is letting go.

BELIEF AND THE NON-ANXIOUS LIFE

To truly create a non-anxious life, you have to *Choose Belief*. I recognize this is where I might lose many of you, but please stay with me. If I don't make my case, you can disregard my perspective here and move on. But my hope is to offer a final portal into the non-anxious life—the foundation that your entire life is anchored to.

Choosing belief comes in two parts: letting go of control and anchoring into the Source. Letting go of control is fairly self-explanatory. You must release the idea that you own your loved ones, should dominate the lives of your kids, employees, clients, or friends, or need to have input regarding all the world's affairs. At the same time, you have to believe you are anchored into something bigger than yourself. Something that operates within you, through you, and beyond you. Something that was before you and that will be after you.

Letting go and anchoring can't work without each other. If you let go of control without anchoring to the Source, you become lost in the wind. You are led around by feelings and political and poetic meanderings. If you try and anchor to the Source, but you don't let go of control, you become part of a long line of destructive religious, political, or ideological madness.

You must choose both.

This is belief.

In the previous chapters, we've discussed things you need to *do*. Actions like choosing freedom, choosing reality, choosing connection, and choosing health and healing. We also took a chapter-long walk through a new way of being: mindful, aware, curious, and intentionally responsive.

In this chapter, we will dig into what may sound like pop-theo-psychological babbling.

Rest assured, it's not.

In fact, it's one of the most profound truths woven into the fabric of existence. A non-anxious life is about vulnerability and surrender in the most cosmic sense.

You're anchoring yourself into something bigger and jumping out of the plane. As former CEO of Google X and best-selling author Mo Gawdat describes it, "Our universe is far too complex to predict. Surrendering oneself to a design that is beyond our ability to grasp is freeing. That freedom is joy."[84]

Most of us, however, try to achieve a non-anxious life by seeking to control every variable in our environment. Unfortunately for many of us, the prevailing cultural wisdom is as direct as it is wrong. We are told: Control is key. Maintaining a tight grip on the steering wheel is the only way to keep everything and everyone in its place.

Many of our society's psychological constructs aim toward self-actualization, to this prevailing moment when we will finally be the center of our own universe. This leads us to a single, inevitable conclusion: You can only rely on and anchor to one thing—

Yourself.

Yet as we have all become more self-actualized, we are being faced with an unmooring truth: the self cannot carry the universe.

---

[84] Mo Gawdat, *Solve for Happy: Engineer Your Path to Joy* (New York: Gallery Books, 2018), 330.

And we are crumbling under the weight. The center does not hold.

A BRIEF HISTORY OF THE BREAKDOWN OF BELIEF

Throughout human history, people have been guided by their tribe, their environment, and their gods. They ate what was available to them on the fringes of the desert, alongside the sea, or on the inland plains. Or they were nomads, moving with the food sources and seasons. They mated with, married, and made family legacies with those in their geographical range. They depended on a higher power, a god or series of gods, to send the rain, dry the land, grow the crops, bring forth food, find a mate, and calm the storms.

But over the past several hundred years, we've taken these jobs from the gods and begun to solve these problems for ourselves. We have millions and millions of dating and mating opportunities—we just swipe right or left. We have avocadoes shipped in from Mexico, fish shipped in from Japan, grain shipped in from Nebraska and Ukraine, and coffee shipped in from Guatemala. These perishable goods are delivered by boats built in China and powered by oil pumped out of the ground in West Texas and the Middle East. We understand weather patterns and, with the help of AI and machine learning, we're improving our ability to predict weather, allowing more and more of us to escape or survive the fires and floods and damaging winds that decimated entire civilizations in previous centuries.

And now we can move. Coast to coast. Internationally. If I don't like my rent in New York, I can move to Kansas. If I don't like Kansas, I can move to Houston. If I am not well in the desert, I will move near the ocean. And yes, I know I'm oversimplifying things like financial resources, family connections, and the costs of moving. On a global scale, billions of people are stuck, hungry, and seeking safety. But chances are, if you're holding this book, you have choices.

Here's my point: Culturally and technologically speaking, we have solved many of the vexing problems that have plagued humanity since the dawn of time.

The accomplishments are truly astounding. We've created possibilities for billions of lives.

And understandably, we've become very arrogant.

We're planning more trips to the moon.[85] Cancer vaccines. Flying cars. Laser-guided missile systems, machine learning, and large-scale, indoor, hydroponic gardening.

And then something like Covid shows up.

Or Dad has a stroke.

Or your neighbor falls and breaks her hip.

One minute Dad is telling jokes on the phone, and the next minute you and your brother are making end-of-life decisions.

---

[85] I'm a believer. We landed on the moon. And the earth is round. And I've seen Bigfoot—but he was just a really hairy buddy I knew in college.

Yesterday you and your neighbor were planning a community garden. Today, you're visiting her in assisted living.

We've achieved some unbelievable advancements. And many more are on the way. But as we tighten our grip on our lives, we're all waking up to a single, terrifying truth:

We control very little of the world around us.

And while we circumvent the Six Daily Choices wheel, our body is keeping the score.

ON A PERSONAL LEVEL

Despite our bluster, our endless pursuit of power and achievement and more, we know this to be true. We are reminded every day.

- When the doctor pulls you and a crisis worker into a small room and says the harrowing words, "There's nothing more we can do." And just like that, he's gone.
- Or when your little daughter wakes you up in the middle of the night with a devastating headache, and several doctors' visits later, someone says the word *cancer*.
- Or when your wife of 18 years meets a guy at work who makes her laugh really, really hard. And he's smart and he's kinda cute. And without warning, she stops coming home.

We don't control much. And the tighter we hang on, the louder our body sounds the alarms.

We can mitigate risk all we want, maximize our protein intake, track our steps, and go to grad school. We can be diligent about weekly date nights, build underground bunkers, and install solar panels on the barn. Many of these things are great—having good health, great relationships, and the absence of deep pain makes our short ride on this planet much more pleasurable. But even when we try and check every variable off the list, we all know how this ride ends. None of us gets out of it alive.

One night while I was in the darkest throes of my anxiety, my wife and I were reading books in bed. I had an epiphany, and like a moron, I shared it right away instead of letting it pass.[86]

I pulled my book down and looked her directly in the eye. "You know, life is the worst . . . Best-case scenario, I'm 95 and you're 94, and it's New Year's Eve. We wait for the clock to strike midnight, we kiss a long, passionate kiss, and then we both fall over dead, and Hank [our son, who was two years old at the time] has to deal with our bodies.

"This is the best-case scenario," I added, "and every other scenario is just a more-awful ending to our inevitable exit from the planet."

Clearly, I wasn't well. My wife was not impressed or amused, and my timing and delivery were awful.

---

[86] This is a common newlywed error. A good rule of thumb is: (a) Have a thought. (b) Start to share it with your new, kind, and unsuspecting wife. (c) Don't.

But I was right.

One day our lives just end. We may be able to prolong life and make the ride more comfortable. But ultimately, we can't control the beginning or the end.

DEATH ANXIETY

And so we're left trying to figure out how to live, knowing this ride involves a one-way ticket. World-renowned psychiatrist, best-selling author, and existential psychologist Dr. Irvin Yalom wrote often on the concept of "death anxiety." The core idea of death anxiety is that people are haunted by the understanding that they will die. In his book *Staring at the Sun*, Yalom writes: "It's not easy to live every moment wholly aware of death. It's like trying to stare the sun in the face: you can stand only so much of it."[87]

The idea of death anxiety, where we step back and take a wide-angle view of our scurrying, chaotic little lives as a way to numb ourselves from our inevitable end, has captivated religious scholars, philosophers, and healing professionals for centuries. Our endless pursuits of more—more power, more money, more prestige, more "being right"—are all just ways of busying ourselves to avoid what comes next.

Our businesses, our religions, and our family trees are sandbag walls we've erected to try to delay the inevitable.

---

[87] Irvin D. Yalom, *Staring at the Sun: Overcoming the Terror of Death* (San Francisco: Jossey-Bass, 2009), 5.

We even go so far, they say, as to personify the universe. We invent deities and gods who listen to our thoughts and judge our actions, we create elaborate after-lives, and with our remaining energy, we seek trophies and accolades and goals. And all this furious action is undertaken for one simple reason: to help turn down our terrified and anxious brains, which are always trying to gently remind us, *Memento mori. Remember you will die.*

Full disclosure . . . I am a practicing Christian who believes in God. I also wholeheartedly understand the existential psychology argument. It makes sense logically and even empirically.

We have logic and empirical thinking to thank for the current state of things. And because we have considered and accomplished so many things, and religions have an admittedly sketchy track record, we've simply thrown the baby out with the bathwater. In more recent world history, we've thrown away belief in a higher power for the worship and belief of logic, rationale, and the scientific method. We worship headlines, sarcasm, and one-sided arguments. We've found great success in grabbing the wheel tighter and tighter, wresting data, efficiencies, and illusory control over so many things.

But what if there's more?

Hold this loosely for a moment: What if a higher power does exist? What if the Source is real?

As renowned attorney Mark Lanier suggests, the measurement of a gallon and the measurement of a yard are not in opposition to one another. They are both valid measurements. But a gallon is not the best way to determine the size of a football field, and a yard is not the best way to measure liquid. Similarly, belief in a higher power doesn't undermine or nullify science, peer-reviewed studies, or inquiry. I like to view such systems as new roads to the same power source. The arc of science leads to belief. And belief circles back to discovery and innovation.

Yes, there are countless peer-review studies, including meta-analysis, suggesting that belief in a higher power helps reduce anxiety and suicide, and strengthens other mental and physical health supports.[88] And there are countless explanations as to the correlative and non-causal nature of these studies. (I'm also certain other studies exist that suggest belief in a higher power makes people more anxious.) But I'm not going to try to measure the height of my room in gallons. These two entrenched positions are simply not in opposition to one another unless a person tries to hold either one too tightly.

So when confronting death anxiety, we must not ask ourselves true-or-false questions. We must look to the center. We must stare directly into the sun by which we have

---

[88] Jalal Poorolajal, Mahmoud Goudarzi, Fatemeh Gohari-Ensaf, and Nahid Darvishi, "Relationship of Religion with Suicidal Ideation, Suicide Plan, Suicide Attempt, and Suicide Death: A Meta-analysis," *Journal of Research in Health Sciences* (Winter 2022), https://www.ncbi.nlm.nih.gov/pmc/articles/PMC9315464/.

lived our pasts, planned our futures, and built our families, our nations, and our beliefs.

We bow before what we put in the center.

This is worship.

And everybody worships.

WORSHIP

In his now-immortalized 2005 graduation speech at Kenyon College, philosopher David Foster Wallace, who is arguably the greatest writer of his generation, delivered a powerful tome entitled "This Is Water." In one of the more classic moments of the speech, Wallace declares,

> Here's something else that's weird but true: in the day-to-day trenches of adult life, there is actually no such thing as atheism. There is no such thing as not worshipping. Everybody worships. The only choice we get is what to worship. And the compelling reason for maybe choosing some sort of god or spiritual-type thing to worship—be it JC or Allah, be it YHWH or the Wiccan Mother Goddess, or the Four Noble Truths, or some inviolable set of ethical principles—is that pretty much anything else you worship will eat you alive. If you worship money and things, if they are where you tap real meaning in life, then you will never have enough, never feel you have enough. . . . Worship your body and beauty and sexual allure and you will always

feel ugly. And when time and age start showing, you will die a million deaths before they finally grieve you. . . . Worship power, you will end up feeling weak and afraid, and you will need ever more power over others to numb you to your own fear. Worship your intellect, being seen as smart, you will end up feeling stupid, a fraud, always on the verge of being found out. But the insidious thing about these forms of worship is . . . that they're unconscious. They are default settings.[89]

When we think of the word *worship*, we generally think of church services or religious ceremonies. But as Wallace suggests, we've entered into a time in history where we have the luxury of *not* bowing before the Great Unknown, begging for mercy and water and food. We worship ourselves.

- We don't have to bow or hope or pray anymore. We just reach out to Amazon Prime.
- We worship work.
- We worship our bodies.

---

[89] I know this is a long quote—thank you for hanging in there and finishing it. I didn't feel I could justifiably paraphrase something this well-written. Wallace's entire speech is a masterpiece and worth a lengthy investment of your time and reflection. David Foster Wallace, "This Is Water," 2005 Kenyon College Commencement Speech (May 21, 2005), https://fs.blog /david-foster-wallace-this-is-water/.

- We worship self-improvement.
- We worship business metrics and data.
- We worship our intellect, our shoes, our haircuts, our net worth.
- We worship our titles, our organic foods, our Instagram followers, how much we bench press, and how many kids we do or don't have.
- We worship our rule books and our religions.
- We worship our kids.
- We worship our pets. Our freedom. Our culture. Our nationality. Our achievements.

In short, we worship what we think will save us.

Notice that almost everything in the above list is based on the word "our." Our world becomes all about us. In a culture built upon self-actualization, inevitably, we end up worshiping ourselves.

Globally, we are realizing that we are not up to the task. The universe does not revolve around us. We are not strong enough to hold it all up. The illusion is falling apart at the seams.

One time my friend SJ and I were surveying the aftermath of a fire that ravaged his ranch. I had been prattling on about weather and science and consequences, though in a few moments of dismayed silence, while SJ and I stood there, he quietly said: "I don't believe there has ever been, in the history of the world, an atheistic agrarian or hunter-gatherer society."

Atheism is a modern privilege.[90] A privilege not born of superior intellectuals and scientists, but of not having to walk out of a tent during a drought and fall to your knees, begging some faceless entity in the heavens, "Please bring rain or my family will die."

A privilege born of being able to turn on the thermostat when the temperature gets too hot or too cold. Or of your insurance company answering the phone after a tornado rips apart your home.

As Wallace says, everybody worships.

THE SEARCH FOR THE ANCHOR

Currently, more people are on anxiety medication than ever before in the history of the world.

Currently, more people are in professional counseling than ever before in the history of the world.

More luxury and wealth exists right now, and is available to more people, than ever before in the history of the world.

And the anxiety levels are in uncharted territory.[91]

We are more anxious than ever. Enter stage left: the Anchor, the Higher Power.

---

[90] Of course, I know there were many ancient writers and thinkers who mocked and laughed at the gods. Here, I'm speaking about wide swaths of civilization.

[91] At least according to what we have on record.

As I mentioned above, full disclosure, I am a Christian. I believe in Jesus and follow his teachings. My belief in God guides my life. I have also spent more than a decade in and around faith-based higher education, working with thousands of students, sitting at the feet of some of the most renowned theologians in the world, and plugging in to local churches in varying degrees. There are thousands of flavors of Christian belief, and millions of people around the world have Christian beliefs that differ from mine. We all read the same Bible, but it speaks to us differently. If I'm perfectly honest, I'm an odd-duck Christian, often falling out of line with many in my community, but still remaining committed to the core, basic tenets, both tangible and mystical.

Billions of other people across the globe have other belief and religious structures. Hindus, Muslims, Deists, and others all believe in something bigger than themselves. I would even argue (and I'm certainly willing to be proven wrong) that Buddhism, though not a theistic religion, is devoted to the collective eternal. Something infinite and ongoing.

I have deep, loving friendships with many thoughtful atheists who do not believe in any sort of deity, but who do believe in the higher power of nature, the endless cycles of death and rebirth, and their own inability to ultimately avoid their role in this cycle.

So hear me say this clearly: I'm not trying to convince you of any particulars. I know what I believe, what my family believes, and I'm at peace.

I am not advocating for a particular religion. Or a particular belief. Or devotion to a lowercase "g" god or an uppercase "G" God. Father Richard Rohr says, "God is always bigger than the boxes we build for God, so we should not waste too much time protecting the boxes."[92]

I'm also not prescribing for you a set of religious rules, regulations, or practices. Religion is people trying to figure out the rules for living under a shared set of values and guidelines. It's always going to be messy. It's always going to be hard. Yes, belief in a higher power has been used for political ends. For societal control. For power structures, abuses, and all sorts of evil. It has also been the source of deep and transformative good.

Science and technology are in that same boat. While they have radically improved our lives for the better, science and technology have been used (and are being used) for political ends, for societal control, war, and personal intrusions of all sorts. Emmy-award winning comedian and writer Jon Stewart explains that science has gotten really good at solving problems—the problems created by science. And science and technology have radically improved our lives in many ways.

All this to say: If we're going to throw rocks, let's be consistent about where we're throwing them (specifically, at who or what). More importantly, I'm saying that to truly create a

---

[92] Richard Rohr, *Everything Belongs: The Gift of Contemplative Prayer* (New York: Crossroad, 2003), 24.

non-anxious life, you have to believe in a transcendent, ever-lasting source. Something bigger than you. As soon as you deeply own how small and miniscule you really are, how brief your life is, and how little power, influence, and control you have . . . you're starting to tie in to the Anchor—the divine that exists beyond us.

And remember: Once you're anchored, belief isn't about holding on tighter. It's about releasing your grip.

Ultimately, you have to let go.

You have to jump.

SARCASM AND PESSIMISM AND THE ILLUSION OF WISDOM

My mentor, Randy Harris, is a monk, a former professor of bioethics and theology, and a pastor. He once told me something deeply profound over enchiladas and tacos: "We live in an age when sarcasm and pessimism so often present as wisdom, while joy and optimism so often show up as insanity."

Cue my nothing-left-to-say-silence.

Holding up the universe is a ton of work. After a while, our hold begins to shake. We get sick, anxious, and exhausted. And when our arms are weakening under the weight of the world, we start looking at our neighbors, who are desperately trying to hold up their worlds.

We point fingers. We make biting comments and sarcastic jokes. We exaggerate and gossip. Debate and yell and scream. We are skeptical of everyone, including doctors, teachers, politicians, religious leaders, and our bosses.

We become untethered agents of chaos. Lighting fires here, throwing grenades there. We point out *their* flaws. We expect *them* to work around our problems and challenges and offenses and anxieties because we can no longer bear the thought of any more discomfort.

Father Rohr says that such people

> are frankly, very difficult to live with. Every one of their ego-boundaries must be defended, negotiated, or worshipped. Their reputation, their needs, their nation, their security, their religion, even their ball-team. They convince themselves that these boundaries are all they have to worry about, 'cause they are the sum total of their identity. You can tell if you've placed a lot of your eggs in these flimsy baskets if you are hurt or offended a lot. You can hardly hurt saints. . . . Eccentric [non-centered] persons, though, are a hurt waiting to happen. In fact, they will create tragedies to make themselves feel alive.[93]

It simply doesn't occur to us to set the bricks and burdens of the world down. But we can. So try doing just that.

Set everything down.

The trauma.

The defending.

---

[93] Rohr, *Everything Belongs*, 25.

The angry demands.

The resolve to always be right.

We have to return to the mystical. To the spiritual. To the mystery.

Of course there will be moments—even seasons—of righteous anger, true fear, and exhaustion. But these cannot be our way of life. We have to back away from a life of poisonous, constant sarcasm and pessimism and begin to seek a higher power who offers truth, freedom, peace, and deep, resounding joy.

Here's the paradox:

You're worthy of being loved. You're enough.
You always will be.
AND you cannot do it on your own.

On your own, you don't have enough to cross the finish line.

You are not, and never will be, strong enough to actualize. To become the center of the universe. Nevertheless, you can make so many choices in and across your life. But you can't hold it all together.

It's both/and. A delicate balancing act of loving ourselves and feeling worthy and participating in our changes and choices—while knowing we need a power source to plug into that is bigger than ourselves.

We don't call our cars broken when they're out of gas. They need to be filled up.

Our phones aren't worthless when they're out of battery. They simply need to be plugged in.

Us too.

LETTING GO

Make no mistake, you are important. You're not a piece of crap. You are loved.

But the center cannot hold.

And this is something to rest in, rather than run around trying to prove.

You're finite. We're all finite. And if we want to finally be free of anxiety, we have to anchor in and let go. We have to believe in a higher power, the ultimate form of connection in which we are never, ever alone.

There's no question you can drastically reduce anxiety by choosing connection, choosing reality, choosing free- dom, choosing mindfulness, and choosing health and heal- ing. This is irrefutable across all layers of insight and fields of knowledge.

But if you want to go all the way to truly live, build, and enjoy the fruits of a non-anxious life, you have to surrender. You must choose belief in something greater than yourself, anchoring deep into the bedrock and fully internalizing that you are worthy of love simply because you have been given the breath of life from the source, God, the creator of the cosmos.

This is not only surrender, this is freedom.

Jump.

CHOOSE BELIEF

Chapter Summary and Next Steps

Summary:

- Belief in God or a higher power is critical to a non-anxious life.
- The idea of self-actualization has failed us. We cannot hold the center of the universe together with our finite minds, bodies, and ideas. We must anchor into a source bigger and more infinite than our own limited sense of understanding.
- Faith and belief are not variables to control. Faith and belief are about anchoring in and letting go.
- While faith and belief are private endeavors, they are communal practices.

Things to Do:

- Find a local faith community, and leave your prejudices and presuppositions at the door. Be curious and attend services for 90 days.
- Begin a practice of prayer and journaling. Seek guidance from a spiritual director or advisor. You can also find many useful ideas for prayer and journaling practices online.
- Write down your thoughts about God or a higher power. What do you believe about God? Is God real? Loving? A myth? Omnipotent?

- Begin seeking ways you can "let go" in your life. Look for places where you have tightened your grip on the world, and consciously release them to God or your higher power.

Ask Yourself:

- Look at your calendar and your budget and ask:
  - What do I worship? My car? My home? My body? Beauty? God? The news? Social media?
  - What gets the lion's share of my time, attention, and resources?
- What do I believe about submitting to God or a higher power?
- What are ways I can improve my relationship with God or a higher power? In what ways am I not ready or willing to do so just yet?

Additional Resources:

- Go to johndelony.com/resources for a list of books, podcasts, and tools to help you start down the path toward a non-anxious life.

CHAPTER 10

THE HARD PATH

I once met with a woman named Alice. She was struggling with whether she should end her marriage of almost two decades. Her husband had abused her, cheated on her, and had continued to treat her with little regard for her safety, dignity, or worth. Her description of the things he did and the things he said to her was enraging.

She deserved so much more.

But Alice could also glimpse what was on the other side of leaving her husband: Constant terror. Financial, food, and shelter insecurity. The kids were in college, and she believed her husband would stop paying their tuition. Alice had nowhere to go, no one to turn to, and yet she could not remain in a marriage that was burying her alive.

As I often do in conversations like this, I asked for her permission to be completely honest. I told Alice that what I was going to say would not be comforting or really even helpful in the immediate sense. But I promised I would tell her the truth.

She exhaled deeply and said, "This is why I reached out to you. For the truth."

I paused for a long, heavy second.

"You have no good choices here, Alice. Despite what anyone would tell you, there's not an easy path forward. Ultimately you have to make one of two incredibly difficult choices: Either stay and continue to be subjected to the violence, belittling, and lack of respect, or risk having to move into a shelter for an unknown period of time until you can come up with a job and money for your own place, your own transportation, and your own food. And your adult kids will have to fend for themselves."

She started sobbing.

"I care about you, Alice," I said gently, "and there is no path forward without pain. So instead of trying to maneuver and avoid and dance around pain like you've been doing for so long, accept that the dancing is over. Now you can look ahead to the path that is right and that leaves you with dignity and respect. Which path is that for you?"

WHEN DISCOMFORT BECAME THE ENEMY

A year or so ago, I read a profound and deeply thought-provoking book titled *The Comfort Crisis* by Michael Easter. I read the entire book in a single sitting, and I immediately handed it to my 12-year-old son for him to read.

The book details the perils of our modern world and an illuminating truth: Our bodies crave hard challenges, learning, boredom, stressors, and moving under load (carrying heavy things). Easter says, "Modern humans may have an unmet need to do what's truly difficult for us. New research shows that depression, anxiety, and feeling like you don't belong can be linked to being untested."[94]

Please don't miss how revolutionary Easter's discovery truly is: Our minds, bodies, and souls crave challenge. Difficulty and discomfort. The gauntlet and the fire.

This changes everything.

As I discussed in chapter 9, in many parts of the world we've solved for hunger. We've solved for housing,[95] for clothing, for shelter, and for transportation. We aren't getting attacked by saber-tooth tigers and Kodiak bears anymore, and our enemies don't regularly invade our homes and communities. Millions of us work sitting down, staring at a screen, and we have climate-controlled homes, cars, and offices. I recently sat inside a giant farming tractor with an air-conditioner, GPS system, and cruise control.

A tractor.

We've made the physical parts of our lives easy and converted the stress from our physical bodies to our minds. And even this is rapidly changing. With the invention of digital libraries, AI, calculators, computer apps, and the explosion

---

[94] Michael Easter, *The Comfort Crisis: Embrace Discomfort to Reclaim Your Wild, Happy, Healthy Self* (New York: Rodale Books, 2021), 40.
[95] Though with housing prices in my hometown of Nashville, that might not be totally true.

of tiny, powerful pocket computers masquerading as phones, we're rapidly losing the need (and thus the ability) to think deeply, to recall and remember, and to perform complex thinking tasks.

We ask Alexa. We just Google it. We type it into whatever version of ChatGPT is out this week. We use the map app on our phone. We Uber instead of walking or riding our bike. We have groceries and ready-made sandwiches brought to our doors with the click of a button.

Overnight, we made life easy. Way, way too easy.

And our bodies are melting underneath us.

On the flip side, there are millions of people who are running themselves, their families, and their legacies into the ground. Now that everything is on demand, we have found ourselves with more free time and fewer threats than ever. And instead of using that time to grow relationally, physically, spiritually, or emotionally, we now work more than ever.

We check our email the second our eyes open in the morning. We work through lunch. We don't even come close to using all our allotted vacation days. We work at home, after dinner, into the night. And we check our phones before we drift off to sleep.

As my friend Ian Simkins says, "If busyness is your drug, rest will feel like stress."

Ouch.

We're over-sanitized, over-informed, over-stimulated and under-rested. We've tried to root out all discomfort, pain, and ugliness, and we've found ourselves sick, less mobile, lacking resilience, easily offended, addicted, dying from diseases of despair. Our bodies are anxious messes, weightless from the lack of true challenges and simultaneously weighed down underneath manufactured "chronic stressors—keeping up with the Joneses, work drama, bills, gossip, that kind of thing. . . . We are now . . . getting done in by ourselves. By the tales we tell ourselves about what we need to achieve and when and why and in relation to whom."[96]

We arrived in hell with good intentions, but it's going to take hard, uncomfortable work to climb our way back out.

TWO PURPOSES

We've discussed the Six Daily Choices for building a non-anxious life. Think of choosing the hard path as the wheel that holds together six spokes. The final piece in the non-anxious life is the choice to intentionally, and whenever possible, incorporate hard things into your life.

On purpose.

Sometimes hard things include exercise, therapy, taking the stairs, moving across the country, and other adventures. Other times the hard path includes saying no, rest and restoration, pursuing solitude, asking for forgiveness, forgiving others, going back to church, changing your mind, and learning something new.

---

[96] Easter, *The Comfort Crisis*, 153.

The pursuit of the hard path serves two powerful purposes.

First, it provides you with daily accomplishments and confidence. Not thin, "You go, girl!" or YOLO confidence. That type of confidence is a sham. It's leftover from the failed self-esteem movement of the '80 and '90s. It leaves people full of rhetoric and "Atta boys!" but with no real experience at steadying their minds, spirits, and bodies.

Choosing to do the challenging path grows new neural pathways, develops muscle and resolve, and proves to your mind, body, and spirit, beyond a shadow of a doubt, that YES, YOU CAN.

Second, a lifetime of choosing to take the difficult path prepares you for moments like Alice was facing. Moments when there are only dark, painful paths forward.

- When you find out your disease is incurable.
- When you realize two years into medical school that this isn't the career for you, and you need to start over.
- When your business folds or your home forecloses.
- When your church splits.
- When you admit to yourself you can't marry your fiancé after all.

In their international bestseller *Ikigai*, Héctor García and Francesc Miralles write, "Sooner or later, we all have to face difficult moments, and the way we do this can make a huge difference to our quality of life. Proper training for our mind, body, and emotional resilience is essential for confronting life's ups and downs."[97]

None of the Six Daily Choices is easy by themselves. Every move forward is a move into the unknown. But with a lifetime of choosing the hard path, you learn you can face the unknown with your shoulders thrown back and your head held high. You will seek the choices that are challenging and dive right in.

Not in an anxious, cocky way.

But in a non-anxious, knowing way.

In our modern world, choosing the hard path is an act of rebellion. It is a thumbing-your-nose at the lazy river that is presently drowning so many people and instead declaring, "I will not go quietly into that good night!"

Remember in chapter 1 when we discussed how avoiding or turning away from anxiety actually reinforces it, making our anxiety even stronger? Well, we've come full circle. After making an entire cycle around the Six Daily Choices wheel, we are choosing to turn and face the alarms.

Choosing the hard path will do that for you. Choosing it is choosing to head into the middle of the storm.

It's about choosing courage, even when you don't know what happens on the other side of your decisions.

It's about the ruthless pursuit of peace on the other side.

---

[97] Héctor García and Francesc Miralles, *Ikigai: The Japanese Secret to a Long and Happy Life* (New York: Penguin Books, 2016), 165.

LIFE *IS* HARD!

There's a meme making the rounds on the internet called "Choose Your Hard." It was written by an unknown author, and it is some variation of the following:

Marriage is hard. Divorce is hard. Choose your hard.

Obesity is hard. Being fit is hard. Choose your hard.

Being in debt is hard. Having control of your finances is hard. Choose your hard.

Clearly communicating your needs is hard. Living a life where no one knows your needs is hard. Choose your hard.

Life is always hard. But we can choose our hard. Pick wisely.

Out of the gate, this sounds equal parts inspiration and bro-science nonsense. I like the sentiment—life is hard either way. Living life 100 pounds overweight is very difficult. It's painful, exhausting, and in some situations, embarrassing and even dangerous. And, losing 100 pounds—altering your entire life and finding the person beneath the weight—is also very difficult. There is no easy path forward. So here, the phrase *Choose your hard* works.

But I didn't choose for my friend to die. And my grandma didn't choose Alzheimer's. And none of us chose the Covid-19 pandemic, the run on toilet paper, or the Nickelback reunion tour. In that sense, telling someone to "Choose your hard" as they're holding the hand of their daughter while she receives chemotherapy is disingenuous and harmful.

To be clear, when I say this, I'm referring to the only things in the world we can control: our thoughts and our actions. I'm calling on us to seek challenges, to lift heavy things, to get control of our anger, and to enter a season of grief when the darkness comes.

And also to reject the comfort crisis of our time. To do the scary, tedious, boring, annoying thing. Over and over and over again. To choose discipline over waiting for motivation.

Just keep showing up each day, showing up to make the choices you need to make for yourself and your future.

This isn't sexy. This generally makes for a terrible social media reel. It's done in the shadows, in the cold and dark of the early morning, under the heat of the unforgiving afternoon sun, in the privacy of counselors' offices and church retreats and back-room Alcoholics Anonymous meetings.

It's admitting that life does end and sitting down with an attorney to get your will done. It's paying off all your debts and duct-taping that old car together because you simply stone-cold refuse to take out a car loan. It's studying online after the kids are in bed to get your GED for the sake of not just job options but because you promised yourself you would.

Sometimes it's facing hard realities. It's almost always choosing optimism and hope.

It is a conscious choice, day in and day out, to choose the hard path.

MIND, BODY, AND SOUL

I have divided choosing the hard path into three sections: mind, body, and soul. In each of these sections, we will explore ways that each of us can choose the challenging path. You will notice that many of the other steps on the non-anxious path are illustrated below. You are choosing the hard path when you get out of debt. Choose love. Choose freedom. Choose health. When you decide to be mindful.

Choosing the hard path is what brings the non-anxious life full circle.

Mind: The balance of curiosity and rest.

Choosing the hard path with your mind involves committing to regularly exploring new ideas and experiences, learning new things, engaging in challenging and supportive relationships, and seeking to find places where you were wrong.

It also means making space for being bored. And stopping our maddening addiction to more data, information, and opinions.

I understand that our technology-infused world curates and spoon-feeds us more information than we could ever possibly hope to consume. Digital platforms learn from us, track us, and spit back at us content from creators and sites they know we will likely engage with. Keep in mind: The creators behind our new information era are not interested in accurate and helpful information that will uplift or teach you. They're concerned with your attention span. This means you will have to be intentional about seeking new sources of information. Expert substacks. Books from trustworthy authors. Podcasts or radio programs from thoughtful individuals or experts. Or my personal favorite: deep, challenging conversations with friends, experts, and people who you know see the world differently than you.

Sometimes this will mean turning off YouTube and taking violin lessons from a real person. Sure, you could learn the one solo, right now, that will impress the girl in your community orchestra. But will you truly learn how to play? Will your mind learn to sync with another person in harmony?

Sometimes this will mean asking people to come over to your house and help you fix your broken swing-set instead of rushing out to buy a new one or calling a handyman. You will learn by doing, alongside friends you trust, and you'll learn new skills, deepen connections, and save a few bucks.

Below are three practices for choosing the way with your mind. None of these are difficult to do in and of themselves, but are in fact very difficult to do, day in and day out.

1) *Write.* You can journal. Keep a diary. Have a gratitude practice. Write fiction, non-fiction, or take extensive notes of podcasts and speakers you enjoy.

The act of writing has a way of crystallizing and distilling what we truly believe on a subject. When I get the ideas out of my head and onto paper, I can work through the ideas until I land on specific and concise thoughts. Or, with a regular journaling practice, you can look back at the things you've written over time and see your progress on a particular topic or issue. I have often looked back on old journals and been encouraged to see how I untangled a thorny issue and came to some resolutions. I've also marveled at my ongoing lack of progress on some issues, having sometimes faced the same questions for years.

The act of writing this book clarified for me some places where I must take immediate and bold action—some of which I'll share in the final chapter. I'd known about these things for some time. Taking the time to write them down was deeply clarifying.

2) *Have a regular practice of engaging in new, challenging ideas.* Don't be afraid of new ideas or judge them prematurely. Instead, head into new ideas, ways of doing life, and approaches to challenging problems with a spirit of curiosity and resolve.

I am a huge believer in Charlie Mungor's wisdom on giving an opinion. He says we should not put forth an opinion on a subject before first knowing our opponent's objections to our opinions better than they do. Before I spout my opinions on electric cars, I'm going to drive one. Talk with people who have owned one for a while. Read about how lithium is mined, how the cars are built, and why someone would never buy one. And only then will I make my opinions known.

3) *Seek intentional periods of time of no new information.* You will choose no screens. No phones. No books or podcasts or headphones. No movies or video games. Just good old-fashioned silence.

You'll be shocked at how loud flapping bird wings are when you're actually listening. You'll also be stunned at how loud the trees are on a breezy day, how silently deer move, and how all your senses are heightened as you start to tune in to the world and those around you.

This time of silence and rest will, at first, feel like a waste of time. It will feel like time you could better spend learning something, reading something, or clicking on something. But it is magic. The time will restore your mind, your spirit, and your body.

Body: The balance of action and rest.

I get it. You don't have time. You're tired. You have no energy. There is no way you're going to start working out because your body can't take more than you're already putting it through.

Maybe this is true.

But probably not.

Michael Easter says, "The truth is, every human body can achieve amazing physical feats when it's forced to."[98] Overtraining is very, very rare. Your body can do so much more than you've given it to do. What's more, we utilize rest days as do-absolutely-nothing days. We sleep in. Eat garbage. Watch countless hours of one-sided documentaries. We sloth it up. And then on Sunday night we feel awful. Our anxiety alarms are blaring like crazy. We are listless and joyless, and we have the entire work week staring us in the face.

---

[98] Easter, *The Comfort Crisis*, 224.

My friend Sal DiStefano of Mind Pump Media told me that he used to have personal-training clients skip workouts because they were low on energy. But then six months later, those same clients would come back because they were running low on energy, and a hard workout gave them more energy than they came dragging into the gym with. Energy begets energy.

I know I discussed this in chapter 8, but it's too important to not revisit. Here's the bottom line: If you want to build a non-anxious life, free from being riddled with anxiety, you have to incorporate movement and exercise into every single day.

Every. Day.

I don't care if it's a 10-minute walk, dance, or jujitsu, lifting heavy weights, cardio, yoga, taking a long walk with your wife or kids, or even a CrossFit WOD . . . but you have to move every single day. Be intentional. Push yourself to go hard when you need to and push yourself to back off when you need to. You're playing a long game here of health, longevity, and non-anxious living. You're not trying to get abs before spring break.

Stick with an actual workout plan for more than five days. Try 30 days without skipping. Keep going. Be disciplined and don't negotiate with yourself. I know there is never a day, unless I am deathly ill, that I can afford to skip movement of some sort.

I also have to be super-focused and even obsessive about my sleep. I have to watch what I eat, especially my caloric intake. I track my calories on a coaching app, and I intermittently track my sleep and heart-rate variability on a Garmin watch.

I sometimes leave parties early. I rarely drink alcohol. I turn the lights down after dark and, once I finish the final edits on this book, I plan to become militant about my phone usage in the evenings. I don't read science or deep-thought books in bed—I only read fiction. I intermittently check in with a nutritionist and a doctor, and I've given my wife full permission to gently ask me if I really want four more pieces of pizza and another helping of queso, or if I'm just bored and jonesing for stimulation. I've learned I need and prefer accountability as opposed to just going it alone.

So here's the plan:

Go see a doctor. If you can afford it, work with a physical therapist. Have your blood work done. Make sure your anxiety is not related to other health issues like hormone levels, heart irregularities, or chemical imbalances in your brain.

I wish there was a one-size-fits-all prescription for everyone when it comes to movement. There is not.

Some weeks you'll need to be intense. Other weeks you'll make do with slow movements, recovery, and mobility. But you'll always move.

Do the first easiest thing you can do and will stick to.

One push-up and one sit-up and then a walk to your mailbox and back without stopping? Do it. And then go again in the evening. Or the following day. And do it again and again and again.

You don't have to run out and spend a bunch of money on a fancy gym membership. You can simply get started by doing what you can, with what you have, wherever you are.

Former Navy Seal and best-selling author Jock Willink recommends having a way to exercise or workout at your home. I fully agree. Over the years, I have collected a hodgepodge of weights and dumbbells and other equipment off internet re-sale sites. I have a nice, *Rocky IV*-style home gym that allows me to get a workout in whenever I have a little time. Or you can simply load up a backpack with heavy things and go for a walk. It's called rucking—which is an old military practice—and it's my latest obsession.

Soul: The connected essence.

When I use the word *soul*, I'm referring to your inner being. The part of you that is in sync with the Higher Power. The part of you that seeks joy, finds beauty, and is moved by connected relationships and creating.

Choosing challenge with your soul is about no longer hating yourself, and instead giving yourself grace. It's about changing the way you talk to yourself, being honest about your past, and respectful and dignified about the future you're creating.

This is about finally writing songs. Finally drafting that new work proposal. Building a flower bed. Restoring that old car. Writing a speech or dreaming up a new business idea. As celebrated music producer Rick Rubin says, "The creative process can have a therapeutic power. It offers a sense of deep connection. A safe place to voice the unspeakable and bare the soul. In these cases, art does not unravel the maker, but makes them whole."[99]

Art and life are not only found in museums or finger paintings or zoos. They're everywhere—even the rocks cry out. Creativity, the act of bringing something into being, is a divine endeavor. It is a way to connect with God. It is love and passionate pursuit mingled together, a quiet meditation practice that no one sees.

So is living well. With others in mind. That's "soul art" too.

It's the neighbor's yard you mow and don't post about on social media.

It's the extraordinary tip you leave the waitress at Waffle House, the thank-you card you send to your child's teacher, or the compassionate way you treat the airline employee when your flight gets canceled.

Choosing the hard path when it comes to your soul is about choosing contentment. Or, as my mentor Randy implored, "Never, ever whine." It's about seeking patience. Learning to be kind. It's about forgiveness and not keeping records of wrongs, because those records only weigh *you* down.

It's also something we practice. I can want to create beautiful melodies on my guitar all day, but I have to practice my scales, all by myself, while my buddies are out having

[99] Rick Rubin, *The Creative Act: A Way of Being* (New York: Penguin Press, 2023), 324.

drinks. Or I can want to be a better therapist, but if I'm not willing to put in the work and give life to new skills, new ways of relating, and new business opportunities, I am not honoring the process.

Choosing the hard path with your soul might include spiritual practices. Religious ceremonies. Connections with friends, neighbors, and loved ones. Or it might mean saying yes to adventures that don't sound fun now, but that you know will leave you uplifted. Or it could be about service. Like building homes for the poor in Haiti. Or working a shift at a food pantry.

It's about finding your purpose. Plugging in. Searching for the good and beautiful things. In his *New York Times* best-selling book *Essentialism*, Greg McKeown encourages us to uncommit, do fewer things with greater excellence, and constantly be on the lookout for things to remove from our lives. Ways to declutter our inner soul.

A few years ago, my friend David and I were talking about our careers. I asked him what his next move was going to be. He was a combat veteran who was working as an IT manager for a local school. I assumed he would try and move up as an administrator or find some other IT job somewhere.

His answer transformed me.

He said, "I'm in my dream job. I'm not gonna ever make a bunch of money, but every day I get to help teachers and students figure out better tools for learning. I feel honored that I get to do my job."

David had peace in his soul.

At the time, such peace had never even occurred to me.

Since my first real job at the age of 21, I'd always looked for the next move. The next promotion. The next raise or title change. I was never still, never satisfied, always looking over my shoulder and over yours. I had no peace in my soul.

Following my conversation with David, I remembered a question a good friend of mine, Dr. Richard Beck, once asked me: "What if we lived our lives as though we could never move? Same churches, same neighborhoods, same homes, same jobs. How would we live our lives differently?"

His question haunted me.

Because I would be more honest about my needs. I'd be more willing to engage in difficult conversations—seek connection—versus just cutting and running. I'd put aside petty differences for the sake of our community. John Ortberg says our souls "become sick when we are divided and conflicted."[100]

Joy, connection, creativity, worship, practice, service. With these endeavors, you are choosing the hard path.

THE NON-ANXIOUS LIFE

Choosing reality is difficult. When we choose reality, we come face-to-face with our failures, our shame, and the parts of our lives we keep hidden from each other and ourselves.

---

[100] John Ortberg, *Soul Keeping: Caring for the Most Important Part of You* (Grand Rapids, MI: Zondervan, 2014), 135.

Choosing connection is about as tough as it gets. It's hard to make friends as an adult. We only get a few chances to have decades-long friends, so the pressure in those rare opportunities can be disheartening.

Choosing freedom is arduous. Ramsey Solutions found it takes about two years for most folks to pay off all their debts. And another seven years to pay off their house. Getting rid of a lifetime's worth of books, gadgets, dusty workout equipment, and piles of children's paintings is gut-wrenching. Admitting I have enough guitars is something I am often unwilling to do. Clearing my calendar, revering time as it flies through my fingers, and having relational, professional, and personal boundaries are some of the most difficult challenges I can experience.

Choosing mindfulness is hard. Exiting a life of reactivity and explosion or shutdown, choosing to enter into a life of intentionality, curiosity, and slower reactions, is demanding.

Choosing health and healing is time-consuming, expensive, can be scary, and may feel selfish. It's the choice to put on my oxygen mask so that I am in position to honor and take care of others. And I often don't have a picture of what "well" even looks like.

Choosing belief is almost impossible. The choice to fire myself from the role of defender and sole provider of the universe and learn, over time, to anchor myself into a higher power is as terrifying as it is illogical.

And *choosing the hard path* toward a non-anxious life is, well, a hard path. You're opting to get to work creating a life your body can thrive in. You're not frantically running around silencing the alarms, but establishing an environment where the alarms only sound off when they are absolutely necessary.

SAFETY IS AN ILLUSION

This is not the easy life. Or the perfect life. Or the free-from-tragedy life. That life does not exist. It's an illusion, sprung from Hollywood screens and the pages of romance novels.

It's the non-anxious life.

The antifragile life.

A defiant, counter-cultural life that chooses patience and joy and kindness over frantic schedules and one more dollar on top of one more dollar.

And dying on the hill when absolutely necessary.

In this life, safety is called out for the illusion it truly is. Because even when it looks like it from the starting line, there are no easy paths.

We have to choose our hard.

NO HARD FEELINGS

The score was 25–8.

We were getting crushed.

And we were an 8–0 team. We didn't get crushed.

But the scoreboard doesn't lie.

Let me back up.

I was a high school geography teacher and an assistant track/cross country coach. As a part of my required responsibilities, I had to pick up a secondary sport to coach, in addition to coaching track.

I was given the sophomore boys basketball team.

These young men were incredible. Me? Not so much.

I knew three things about basketball: (1) If you shot from far away, you got three points. (2) If you hit or tackled someone, they got a free shot. (3) If I yelled, "Time out!" everyone stopped. This was particularly cool when games were getting out of control or when one of my players needed to use the bathroom.

Right after cross country season, I was handed a bus, key, and a team of 13 young men. The head basketball coaches did their best to teach me a few offensive plays, inbounds passes, practice drills, and the like. And the players on my team were so gifted, I didn't need much else.

We traveled across the city of Houston, a roving band of brothers, knocking out sophomore team after sophomore team. The boys were having a blast.

I started getting cocky.

Until I yelled, "Time out!" when we were down 25–8.

I was a hot-headed 21-year-old, always pacing the sidelines like I'd seen college coaches do during March Madness. And in my mind at least, the stakes were similarly high.

After the referee blew his whistle, stopping play, our team huddled up. I was hollering, scribbling hieroglyphics on my clipboard, and otherwise making a scene.

"RUN THE OFFENSE! IT'S A SIMPLE MOTION OFFENSE, MEN! . . . PASS AND SCREEN AWAY! PASS AND SCREEN AWAY! WHY IS THIS SO HARD?"

I kept hollering about their failing effort, their lack of heart and desire, and their inability to run the offense. Until Marquis spoke up.

"Coach . . . it's not gonna work."

I lost it.

"WHAT DO YOU MEAN, IT'S NOT GOING TO WORK?!" I bellowed.

Marquis looked up, exasperated, and raised his voice

back. "Our offense isn't going to work! It's a man-to-man offense and they're runnin' a zone."

Uh-oh.

"What do you mean they're running a zone?"

"COACH! They're running a zone! We're trying to pass and screen away but they not movin'."

I was thrust into a fork in the road. I could go left or right, but standing still was not an option.

All my players were looking at me, and the ref was walking over to us to resume the game.

I took a deep breath and, without warning, a smile spread across my face.

"What's a zone?" I asked.

Everybody's eyes grew as big as tennis balls.

"Hurry! What's a zone?"

"Are you serious?" Marquis asked. "It's when they don't move. They just guard a space, not a person."

"They just guard a space? That's the dumbest thing I've ever heard!"

"Coach, are you serious?"

I started laughing.

The ref blew the whistle, signaling the start of play. They looked at each other and began chuckling to themselves.

"Do your best boys. Y'all got this!" I laughed as I sat down on the bench.

I coached them the best I could for the rest of the game, and we got blown out.

I was embarrassed—but my team and I crossed into a new level of vulnerability and trust that night.

I was the coach . . . and I didn't know the answer.

I was the expert they were all looking up to . . . and I didn't know what to say next. It was my job to be living this out so that when we ran into roadblocks, I could lead them on the path forward.

I was supposed to know.

TELLING THE TRUTH

Writing this book has been the hardest project I've ever undertaken. I've written two previous books, two dissertations, and countless academic and administrative projects. I've been a senior leader of multiple organizations, and I'm married and raising two kids.

But this project pushed me to my brink.

I realized about halfway through writing that I was not living these things out.

I have two PhDs and I put myself out there as an expert on anxiety, relationships, and mental-health issues, and I realized I was living a very anxious life.

Old habits had snuck back up on me.

Skipping sleep.

Constantly scrolling on my phone.

Reading books to avoid family time.

Avoiding some childhood issues that I needed to deal with.

A house, car, and work area full of clutter. Papers, gadgets, accessories, and general garbage.

I was late to everything. Again.

I ate garbage, and I tried to work it all off with mayhem workouts at crazy hours of the day and night.

I hadn't meditated in months, and I'd left my Cold-Tub empty, my son wondering if he was the reason I was so grumpy, and my wife holding together a household while I traveled the country as the so-called expert.

I'd become so jaded with faith and church and politics and belief that I'd found myself checked out in a way I hadn't been in years.

Unbelievably, I'd found myself lonely again. I've got great workmates, good friends in other states, church comrades, and some new buddies I've met along the way. But if I was honest, truly honest, my friend and colleague's assessment of me was poignantly on target:

I am very hard to be friends with.

Ugh.

Trappist monk Thomas Merton wrote in his poem "The Inner Law":

> He who is controlled by objects
> Loses possession of his inner self:
> If he no longer values himself,
> How can he value others?
> If he no longer values others,
> He is abandoned.[101]

---

[101] Thomas Merton, *The Way of Chuang Tzu* (New York: New Directions, 1965), 136.

This was me. Except that, unlike my time as a basketball coach, I actually knew the answers.

Reading and researching wasn't the challenge. I just wasn't living what I knew. And so, halfway through this book, the writing took on a highly personal aim. The engine began humming, and the book took on an entirely different life.

It was no longer about me talking *at you*, the reader, telling YOU how to choose and live a non-anxious life. This book was about me walking *with you*—all of us seeking to get our lives back.

About me going back to the well and drawing up fresh water to drink and making sure there was enough to go around.

About us all getting back up on our horses and creating non-anxious lives for ourselves.

NO HARD FEELINGS

As I write this chapter, I've dug in deep on choosing reality. I've taken stock of my life, warts and all. It's been tough and challenging, but here's where I'm headed:

I have a counseling appointment scheduled. I've transformed my workouts and I've made health and healing a priority.

I'm working closely with my team to put some breathing room in my calendar, in my personal time, and at home. I don't owe anyone anything, and my wife and I are committed to a life of freedom from external influences.

I've rededicated myself to eating healthy, to getting deep, rich sleep, and to keeping soul-sucking electronics out of my living room and my bedroom.

I've begun hanging out again, and I've got regular lunch meetings and breakfasts and concerts on the calendar moving forward.

I am meditating every day, and I'm clearing away the academic, political, and cultural madness surrounding what I truly believe and am anchored to.

And that's only the beginning.

But I'm not telling you this to brag or in any way communicate I have everything all together. I'm telling you this because I know, firsthand, how hard it is. And if I can fall, with all my opportunities, resources, and the letters after my name, anyone can.

The moment any of us thinks we've arrived, the dragons show up. As soon as we think we've figured it out in our parenting, our marriages, our eating plans, and our businesses, things will go sideways.

Please hear me loud and clear:

The Six Daily Choices are hard.

They will be for the rest of our lives.

There is simply no way around them. And even if we could go around them, we wouldn't want to.

Because as exhausting as the hard path is, it gets you to the hope.

Brené Brown says, "Hope is a combination of setting goals,

having the tenacity and perseverance to pursue them, and believing in our own abilities. Hope is Plan B."[102]

The anxious mayhem we were living was our Plan A.

It has failed.

So it's time for Plan B.

It's time for hope.

I'm done being a victim.

I'm done thinking more "stuff" will make me happy.

I'm done with unhealthy relationships and putting my family third and fourth in my life.

The ship has turned.

And yours can too.

Ryan Holiday says it this way: "Courage is the management of and the triumph over fear. It's the decision . . . to take ownership, to assert agency, over a situation, over yourself, over the fate that everyone else has resigned themselves to. *We can curse the darkness, or we can light a candle.*"[103]

It's time to turn on all the lights.

Be courageous.

And start lighting candles.

Choose Reality

Choose Connection

---

[102] Brené Brown, *Daring Greatly: How the Courage to Be Vulnerable Transforms the Way We Live, Love, Parent, and Lead* (New York: Avery, 2012), 240.

[103] Ryan Holiday, *Courage Is Calling: Fortune Favors the Brave,* (New York: Portfolio/Penguin, 2021), 84, emphasis added.

Choose Freedom
Choose Mindfulness
Choose Health and Healing
Choose Belief

This is the way to the non-anxious life.

Whichever choices you're focused on, just keep going. When you choose the hard path of reality, freedom, peace, and love, own it and don't give up. Because like the Avett Brothers sing, hard feelings "haven't done much good for anyone."[104]

If you open your eyes, you'll realize there are millions of folks, just like you, choosing daily to do things differently.

I'd love for you to join us.

---

[104] Scott Avett, Timothy Avett, and Robert Crawford, "No Hard Feelings" (2016).

ACKNOWLEDGMENTS

Sheila, Hank, and Josephine: Not a single page of this books exists without you. You are my adventure, my reason, my hope, and my loves. Hank—I am so, so proud of you. Josephine—I am so, so proud of you too. Sheila—thank you for believing in me.

I am but a vapor without you three. Thank you for loving me and for never giving up on me. I am the luckiest man alive.

Dave Ramsey: You continue to be my coach, mentor, and friend. Thank you for your wisdom, your hospitality, and your generosity. What a ride . . .

Cody Bennett: Thank you for your friendship, your world-class ideas, and your willingness to stand toe-to-toe and fight for the best end result. Everything about this project is better because of your involvement.

Rachel Sims and Eva Daniel: Thank you for the last-minute read-throughs, your insights, ideas, and overall brilliance. Rachel—thank you for the Choices. You two are the best of the best.

Preston Cannon: You are the best book publisher in the world. You are an even more incredible man, husband, and father. I know I'm tough to work with during the writing season—again, thank you for never giving up on me.

Kris Bearss: The editor of all editors! Thank you for walking alongside me every step of the way of this project. I'm so grateful for your expertise and late-night phone calls, your relentless drive to love and honor the reader, and most of all, your friendship. You pushed, supported, and cheered me on—and this project is all the better for it (I am too!).

Rick Prall: Thank you for your tireless efforts to keep me on the right track and to take care of the million citation details.

Daniel Ramsey, Jeremy Breland, Suzanne Simms, and Jen Sievertsen: Your input, ideas, and willingness to fight for the strongest book possible made this entire project better than I ever thought it could be. Thank you for your insights, your wisdom, and your friendship.

Big thanks to: Alex and Tracy Pearl; Drs. Steve and Lynn Jennings; Dr. Michael Gomez; Dr. Layne Norton; Joshua, Ryan, and TK of The Minimalists; Sal, Adam, Justin, and Doug of Mind Pump; Will Guidara; Jade Simmons; Shawn Ryan; Dawn Madsen; Link Blevins; Dr. Andy Young; Dr. Janet Hicks; Dr. Beth Robinson; Dr. Bret Hendricks; Dr. aretha marbley; Dr. Loretta Bradley; Dr. Ian Lertora; Holly Cook; SJ Dalhstrom; Wes and Rachel Freitas; JP and Beth Conway; and Dustin Benham.

Mom, Dad, and Brother and Sister Delony; and Jim, Shirley, Justin, and Leslie Brown.

ACKNOWLEDGMENTS

Kelly, Jenna, Ben, Nate, Andrew, Sarah, and Joe: Y'all listened to this material for more than a year. Thank you for helping me sharpen it, grind it down, and make it come alive.

Seth Farmer, Riley Clark, Chris Carrico, Connor Bowser, Bryan Amerine, Tara Astafan, John Smith, Weylon Smith, Brian Horvath, Cory Mabry, Jasmine Cannady, Julia Calvert, Carlee Francis, Samantha Ellis, Megan McConnell, and Tim Scee: You are the most talented group of artists and teammates ever assembled. Thank you for making everything better than real life . . . and thank you for always making sure I'm where I need to be.

Rachel, Ken, Jade, George, and Eddie: Ride or die. Thanks for letting me be in the gang.

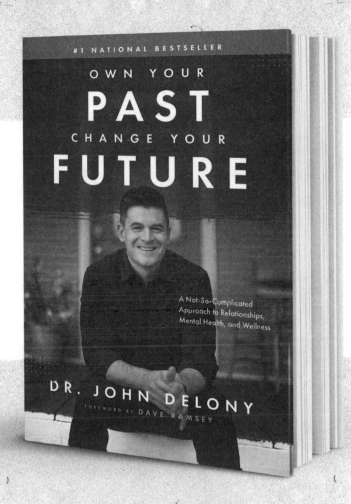

The Greatest Mental Health Podcast Ever

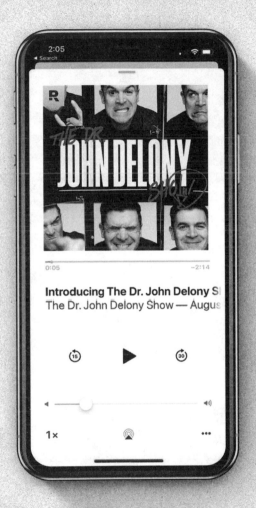

The Dr. John Delony Show is a caller-driven show that helps you find the answers to questions about mental health, wellness, relationships, and more.

johndelony.com